Metabolic Acidosis

Donald E. Wesson

Editor

Metabolic Acidosis

A Guide to Clinical Assessment
and Management

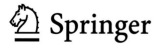 Springer

Editor
Donald E. Wesson, MD, MBA
Baylor Scott and White Health
Department of Internal Medicine
Texas A&M Health Sciences Center College of Medicine
Temple, TX, USA

ISBN 978-1-4939-3461-4   ISBN 978-1-4939-3463-8   (eBook)
DOI 10.1007/978-1-4939-3463-8

Library of Congress Control Number: 2015954357

Printed on acid-free paper

This Springer imprint is published by Springer Nature
The registered company is Springer Science+Business Media LLC New York

Preface

As delivery of healthcare transitions from a focus on episodes of care delivery to restore health (i.e., "sick" care) to maintaining health of populations (i.e., "population health"), it will become increasingly important to delegate responsibility for care of conditions that threaten health to providers who are more proximal to individuals receiving that care. Many medical conditions for which routine care has been provided by subspecialists and specialists must have this routine care delegated to primary care providers, with possible guidance from subspecialists and specialists, in evolving models of population health. The latter strategy better leverages limited provider resources and allows for better opportunities for provider-patient engagement with the potential for enhanced patient and public outcomes.

Metabolic acidosis is a surprisingly common disorder, in both its acute and chronic forms, that threatens overall patient and public health and is a candidate condition for management by primary care providers. Because metabolic acidosis in its chronic and mild forms is typically well compensated by body systems and therefore tolerated reasonably well, it was historically thought to have few if any major untoward effects. By contrast, more recent studies detailed herein show metabolic acidosis to have many consequential untoward effects that can reduce the quality and even the length of life of its sufferers. Widening the army of providers to include primary care providers who can identify and manage this common disorder holds promise to limit its devastating effects.

The expert contributors to this book iteratively build toward recommended management of metabolic acidosis by beginning with a basic understanding of the physiology that under most circumstances precludes development of metabolic acidosis and the reasons for the breakdown or overwhelming of these protective mechanisms. They then establish a basic understanding of the pathophysiology of metabolic acidosis to help identify its presence within the sometimes complicated context of the multiple disease processes that can cause it. These experts then develop management strategies based on this physiology and pathophysiology. This recommended management includes not only that carried out by the healthcare provider but that that can be done by the individual patient, including dietary management.

I am indebted to the expert contributors to this book that is designed to be a guide for primary care providers in managing patients with metabolic acidosis and for the education of the wide spectrum of healthcare professional trainees. I am also thankful to the countless patients who volunteered their participation in studies that have enhanced our understanding of their medical conditions, including metabolic acidosis, which has helped in the design of increasingly better management strategies for this common disorder. Their contribution and the work of countless experts, including those contributing this book, have improved the management of metabolic acidosis and limited its devastating consequences. Our hope is that this book will help frontline providers leverage this understanding to further limit the untoward consequences of metabolic acidosis.

Temple, TX, USA   Donald E. Wesson, MD, MBA

Contents

Contributors

Matthew K. Abramowitz, M.D., M.S. Division of Nephrology, Department of Medicine, Albert Einstein College of Medicine, Bronx, NY, USA

Department of Epidemiology & Population Health, Albert Einstein College of Medicine, Bronx, NY, USA

Afolarin Amodu, M.D., M.P.H. Division of Nephrology, Department of Medicine, Albert Einstein College of Medicine, Bronx, NY, USA

Daniel Batlle, M.D. Division of Nephrology and Hypertension, Northwestern University Feinberg School of Medicine, Chicago, IL, USA

Thomas D. DuBose Jr., M.D., M.A.C.P., F.A.S.N. Section on General Internal Medicine, Wake Forest School of Medicine, Winston Salem, NC, USA

Lynda Frassetto, M.D. Department of Medicine, University of California San Francisco, San Francisco, CA, USA

Nimrit Goraya, M.D. Baylor Scott and White Health, Texas A&M Health Sciences Center College of Medicine, Temple, TX, USA

Csaba P. Kovesdy, M.D. Division of Nephrology, University of Tennessee Health Science Center, Memphis, TN, USA

Jeffrey A. Kraut, M.D. Division of Nephrology, VHAGLA Healthcare System, Los Angeles, CA, USA

Melvin E. Laski, M.D. Department of Internal Medicine, Texas Tech University Health Sciences Center, Lubbock, TX, USA

Glenn T. Nagami, M.D. Medicine and Research Services, VA Greater Los Angeles Healthcare System, Los Angeles, CA, USA

Department of Medicine, David Geffen School of Medicine at UCLA, Los Angeles, CA, USA

Nitin Relia, M.D. Division of Nephrology and Hypertension, Northwestern University Feinberg School of Medicine, Chicago, IL, USA

Khurram Saleem, M.D. Department of Nephrology, Northwestern Memorial Hospital, Chicago, IL, USA

Donald E. Wesson, M.D., M.B.A. Baylor Scott and White Health, Department of Internal Medicine, Texas A&M Health Sciences Center College of Medicine, Temple, TX, USA

Chapter 1
Overview of Acid–Base Physiology

Nimrit Goraya and Donald E. Wesson

Introduction

Optimal cell and tissue function requires that hydrogen ion (H⁺) concentration of body fluids be maintained in a relatively narrow range. Pure or "neutral" H_2O has $[H^+] = 100$ nM or 100×10^{-9} M $= 10^{-7}$ M $= 10^{-7}$ mol/L. Because pH of an aqueous solution is its negative log in moles/liter, pure or "neutral" H_2O has pH $= 7.00$. Under normal steady-state conditions, multiple and redundant systems described subsequently maintain human extracellular fluid [ECF] in a slightly alkaline (compared to pure H_2O), remarkably narrow range of 35–45 nM (pH 7.46–7.35). Otherwise healthy humans can tolerate acute $[H^+]$ levels between 16 and 160 nM (pH 7.8–6.8) but body systems work to return $[H^+]$ closer to the normal value of 40 nM (pH = 7.4) for optimal cell and tissue function. Because $[H^+]$ is determined by the ratio of PCO_2/HCO_3 [1], $[H^+]$ is maintained within this narrow range and/or returned toward normal by manipulation of the respiratory component (PCO_2) in the numerator (CO_2 gas yields H⁺ when dissolved in aqueous solution) and the metabolic component (HCO_3) in the denominator.

An acidosis is a *process* in which body fluids experience a net increase in $[H^+]$ or loss of base. Conversely, an alkalosis is a *process* in which body fluids experience a net decrease in $[H^+]$ or increase in base. Note that these definitions do not indicate what is the ambient $[H^+]$ but only the directional $[H^+]$ change that are the dynamic processes of acidosis and alkalosis. The ambient $[H^+]$ of ECF is described by the

N. Goraya, M.D.
Baylor Scott and White Health, Texas A&M Health Sciences Center College of Medicine, 2401 South 31st Street, Temple, TX 76508, USA
e-mail: ngoraya@sw.org

D.E. Wesson, M.D., M.B.A. (✉)
Baylor Scott and White Health, Department of Internal Medicine, Texas A&M Health Sciences Center College of Medicine, 2401 South 31st Street, Temple, TX 76508, USA
e-mail: dwesson@sw.org

© Springer Science+Business Media New York 2016
D.E. Wesson (ed.), *Metabolic Acidosis*, DOI 10.1007/978-1-4939-3463-8_1

states of acidemia (higher than normal [H⁺]) and alkalemia (lower than normal [H⁺]). Thus, a patient might have a process of acidosis in the setting of the state of alkalemia if he/she has a mixed acid–base disorder. When the process of acidosis is caused by an increase in the respiratory (PCO_2) component in the numerator of the PCO_2/HCO_3 ratio, the process is called respiratory acidosis. When the process of acidosis is caused by a decrease in the metabolic (HCO_3) component of the ratio, the process is called metabolic acidosis, the topic of this book.

Metabolic acidosis is therefore characterized by a primary (i.e., initial event, not a secondary or responding event) decrease in serum [HCO_3]. Remembering that [H⁺] is determined by the PCO_2/HCO_3 ratio, it is evident that the body can ameliorate the resulting increase in the ambient [H⁺] in response to the decrease in [HCO_3] by concomitantly lowering PCO_2. This is exactly what happens under circumstances of normally functioning lungs and is called a physiologic (in this case, respiratory) response to metabolic acidosis. Note that this respiratory response is not a "compensatory respiratory alkalosis" because calling it a respiratory alkalosis indicates a pathologic increase in ventilation, which the described circumstance is not. What has been described is a normal response of normally functioning lungs to a metabolic acidosis. The acid–base disturbance described is properly called a metabolic acidosis with a respiratory response. Consequently, metabolic acidosis as a single (not part of a mixed) disorder is characterized by a decrease in serum [HCO_3] and a decrease in blood PCO_2. Disturbances of acid–base balance are commonly recognized through the described changes in serum and blood acid–base parameters although clinicians must also employ data obtained from history and physical exam to make an accurate acid–base diagnosis.

Maintenance of Normal Acid–Base Homeostasis

Maintenance of normal, steady-state systemic acid–base status involves the elegant integration of physiologic mechanisms such as extra- and intracellular buffering processes and collaborative actions of a number of organs including the kidney, liver, lung, gastrointestinal tract, and skeleton. Recognizing these defense mechanisms reminds clinicians that when metabolic acidosis becomes evident, in part through the described changes in serum/blood acid–base parameters, the net [H⁺] increase has exceeded the capacity of (1) body buffers to prevent a decrease in serum [HCO_3]; and/or (2) organ(s) that ordinarily defend against an increase in [H⁺] or restore it to normal, at least temporarily. Recognition of underlying metabolic acidosis or any other acid–base disorder can lead clinicians to the diagnosis of specific diseases that might not be immediately evident. For example, metabolic acidosis in a patient might be due to lactic acidosis that is caused by underlying sepsis. On the other hand, metabolic acidosis itself, particularly in its chronic form, is associated with a number of metabolic derangements that adversely affect overall health. Consequently, if the cause for the metabolic acidosis cannot be removed, metabolic acidosis must be treated in an effort to prevent or mitigate its untoward effects.

In general, the larger the H+ challenge to systemic acid–base, including intake of diet components that increase intrinsic H+ production, the greater the decrease in ambient serum [HCO$_3$] [2]. Nevertheless, large increases in dietary H+ intake elicit quantitatively small decreases in serum pH and serum [HCO$_3$] (and vice versa) and changes in both in response to increased dietary H+ typically fall within the normal range for each [2]. Consequently, individuals with normal glomerular filtration rate (GFR) who ingest a diet of very high H+ content will typically have serum/blood acid–base parameters that fall within the normal range, even with an apparent net increase in ECF [H+] [2]. These data attest to the effectiveness of normal physiologic processes to protect against large changes in serum acid–base parameters in response to major increases (or decreases) in dietary H+. On the other hand, the same dramatic increase in dietary H+ in individuals with reduced GFR might yield changes in acid–base parameters that are consistent with metabolic acidosis [3], particularly in elderly individuals whose serum creatinine might be reflective of much lower GFR than in younger individuals with the same creatinine [4].

Human studies show that kidney H+ excretion increases in response to an increase in dietary H+ but that the increment in kidney H+ excretion is less than the increment in dietary H+, consistent with net H+ retention [5]. Because even substantial increments of dietary H+ are typically accompanied by only minor decreases in serum [HCO$_3$] [2] that remain stable despite continuation of the increment in dietary H+ [5, 6], it appears that most of this retained H+ titrates body buffers. In addition, patients with reduced GFR are more likely to develop metabolic acidosis in response to an increment in dietary H+ than are those with normal GFR [3]. Consequently, patients with reduced GFR might be at higher risk for H+ retention while eating the high dietary H+ that is typical of diets in industrialized societies [7]. Indeed, patients with even modestly reduced estimated GFR (eGFR) appear to have H+ retention [8]. At least some of this retained H+ is buffered by bone [5] which is a large source of calcium carbonate and dibasic phosphate buffers. Because bone buffering of retained H+ consumes its finite mineral content, bone may not to be the sole buffer source for what appears to be ongoing H+ retention. Consequently other, as yet unidentified, buffer sources might also contribute. Future studies will determine if patients without metabolic acidosis by serum/blood acid–base parameters but who appear to have H+ retention should be candidates for treatment, including with dietary H+ reduction.

The signal(s) that tell kidneys to increase urine H+ excretion when GFR is reduced in the absence of metabolic acidosis are not clear. Animals with partial nephrectomy sufficient to reduce GFR but not sufficient to be associated with metabolic acidosis have tissue H+ retention despite having plasma acid–base parameters not different from control (sham) animals [9, 10] similar to patients with reduced GFR but no metabolic acidosis [8]. Consequently, acid–base parameters in fluid compartments other than plasma might signal kidney responses to retain H+ in the setting of normal plasma acid–base parameters. Candidate compartments include interstitial fluid as suggested by animal studies [9–11] measured by specific pH sensors like GPR4 [12]. Other or additional signals might be the degree of titration of body buffers. Further studies will be required to better answer this important question.

Systemic and Renal Acid–Base Homeostasis

Body systems can ameliorate the effect of added H^+ to increase ECF $[H^+]$ (or to decrease pH) and decrease serum $[HCO_3]$ by (1) employing the HCO_3/H_2CO_3 buffer system; (2) binding the added H^+ to non-HCO_3 buffers in both the extra- and intracellular fluid; and (3) excretion from the body, predominantly by the kidney through the urine.

HCO_3/H_2CO_3 Buffer System Adding H^+ to body fluids containing HCO_3, leads to the following reaction:

$$H^+ + HCO_3 \rightarrow H_2CO_3 \rightarrow H_2O + CO_2$$
$$- (CO_2 \text{ gas is excreted from the body by the lungs})$$

Consequently, the added H^+ is effectively removed from the blood as CO_2 gas that would otherwise yield H^+ (in a reversal of the above equation) if it were to accumulate. This rapidly responsive system works well to minimize the increase in $[H^+]$ (or decrease in pH) that would otherwise occur in the absence of this elegant system. The price paid is a reduction in ECF $[HCO_3]$ that must be regenerated through H^+ excretion by the kidney (see below).

Non-HCO_3 Buffers It is "free" in solution or "unbound" H^+ that determines the acid–base effect on cell and tissue function. Binding H^+ to buffers takes it out of solution and greatly diminishes its untoward effect on cells and tissues. The major non-HCO_3 ECF buffers are hemoglobin and albumin whereas phosphate ion and anionic proteins are the major non-HCO_3 intracellular buffers. Quantitatively, most H^+ binding to non-HCO_3 buffers occurs intracellularly [13]. Bone calcium carbonate and dibasic phosphate are important buffers for both acute and chronic metabolic acidosis in patients [5].

H^+ Excretion The kidney is the main contributor to excretion of metabolically produced fixed H^+. Diets of individuals in industrialized societies typically contain the equivalent of 60–100 mmol of H^+ daily. To excrete 100 mmol of H^+ in the typical daily urine volume of 1 L would require excreted urine to have a $[H^+] = 100$ mmol/L $= 100 \times 10^{-3}$ M $= 10^{-1}$ M $=$ pH of 1.0 (remember that pH is the negative log of the $[H^+]$ in mol/L). Because humans are unable to reduce urine pH below 4.0 ($=[H^+]$ of 10^{-4} M) which is equal to $[H^+]$ of 0.1 mM $= 0.1$ mmol/L, to excrete 100 mmol of H^+ in urine with pH 4.0 would require 100 mmol/0.1 mmol/L $= 1000$ L of urine! Hence, kidneys excrete ingested and metabolically produced fixed H^+ predominantly as H^+ bound to buffers, not as free H^+ in solution. Quantitatively, ammonium $[NH_4^+$ from $NH_3 + H^+]$ is the most important urine buffer followed by "titratable acidity," most of the latter being phosphate ($HPO_4 = \rightarrow H_2PO_4^-$).

Organ Contributors to Systemic Acid–Base Status

Liver Metabolism of ingested amino acids by the liver yields H^+, HCO_3, or neither, depending on the nature of the amino acids ingested. The typical diet of those living in industrialized societies yields net H^+ when metabolized [7] so kidneys of these individuals are typically excreting H^+, mostly in the form of NH_4^+ and titratable acidity. The liver is a major provider of glutamine, the source of most NH_4^+ used for H^+ excretion in the urine as described.

Lungs Cellular metabolism produces about 15,000 mmol of CO_2 daily that as indicated earlier, yields H^+ when dissolved in aqueous solution as follows:

$$CO_2 + H_2O \rightarrow H_2CO_3 \rightarrow HCO_3 + H^+$$

The HCO_3 might leave ECF or be buffered in the extra- or intracellular fluid, leaving H^+. Fortunately, ECF flowing through the lungs makes this an "open" system for CO_2 gas to be excreted rather than be retained if this were a closed system, thereby avoiding H^+ retention.

Gut Dietary components that when metabolized impact system acid–base status are absorbed through the gastrointestinal tract. These components include amino acids as described but also organic anions derived from bacterial metabolism of ingested carbohydrates, protein, and fat. Absorbed organic anions constitute potential base because they can be metabolized by the liver to yield HCO_3. Organic acids might also be retained in the gut to titrate HCO_3 to H_2O and CO_2, thereby reducing gut HCO_3 that might be absorbed into ECF. Finally, these organic acids might be excreted from the body in the stool, representing a loss of potential HCO_3.

Bone Both acute and chronic metabolic acidosis are accompanied by an increase in urine calcium excretion [14], reflecting loss of calcium and its accompanying base from bone [15].

Kidney As indicated earlier, H^+ produced from metabolism consumes body fluid HCO_3 and therefore its buffering capacity, particularly in ECF. Consequently, HCO_3 filtered into kidney tubules must not only be reabsorbed (recovered) as completely as possible to minimize its loss from the body, new HCO_3 must be regenerated to replace that which was consumed as described. These are the two main kidney responsibilities with respect to maintenance of acid–base homeostasis. Each task is accomplished by H^+ secretion from kidney tubule cells into the tubule lumen. When there is a high amount of HCO_3 in the tubule lumen as is the case in the proximal tubule, secreted H^+ titrates luminal HCO_3 to CO_2 and H_2O as described and CO_2 gas diffuses into the cell and is reconstituted to HCO_3 by the enzyme carbonic anhydrase. Reconstituted HCO_3 is transported across basolateral membranes of tubule cells to return to the systemic circulation. When the tubule content of HCO_3 is low as in the distal nephron, most secreted H^+ titrates non-HCO_3 buffers that are excreted in the urine, mostly as NH_4^+ and titratable acidity. With exit of secreted H^+ from the body as described, the distal nephron cell can form new HCO_3 from intracellular CO_2 using carbonic anhydrase and the newly synthesized HCO_3 can then be transported from the cell into the systemic circulation as described. The latter process is referred to as net acid excretion because it excretes the net acid that was produced and/or exogenously added. Net acid excretion is equal in amount to HCO_3 regeneration. Increments in net acid excretion promoted by increments in dietary H^+ intake are mediated mostly by an increase in urine NH_4^+ excretion.

References

1. Kassirer JP, Bleich HL. Rapid estimation of plasma carbonate tension from pH and total carbon dioxide content. N Engl J Med. 1965;272:1067.
2. Kurtz I, Maher T, Hulter HN, et al. Effect of diet on plasma acid–base composition in normal humans. Kidney Int. 1983;24:670–80.
3. Adeva MM, Souto G. Diet-induced metabolic acidosis. Clin Nutr. 2011;30:416–21.
4. Frassetto LA, Todd K, Morris Jr RC, Sebastian A. Estimation of net endogenous noncarbonic acid production in humans from diet potassium and protein contents. Am J Clin Nutr. 1998;68:576–83.
5. Lemann Jr J, Bushinsky DA, Hamm LL. Bone buffering of acid and base in humans. Am J Physiol. 2003;285:F811–32.
6. Goodman AD, Lemann C, Lennon EJ, et al. Production, excretion and net balance of fixed acids in patients with renal acidosis. J Clin Invest. 1965;44:495–506.
7. Remer T. Influence of nutrition on acid–base balance-metabolic aspects. Eur J Nutr. 2001;40:214–20.
8. Wesson DE, Simoni J, Broglio K, Sheather S. Acid retention accompanies reduced GFR in humans and increases plasma levels of endothelin and aldosterone. Am J Physiol Renal Physiol. 2011;300:F830–7.
9. Wesson DE, Simoni J. Increased tissue acid mediates progressive GFR decline in animals with reduced nephron mass. Kidney Int. 2009;75:929–35.
10. Wesson DE, Simoni J. Acid retention during kidney failure induces endothelin and aldosterone production which lead to progressive GFR decline, a situation ameliorated by alkali diet. Kidney Int. 2010;78:1128–35.
11. Wesson DE. Dietary acid increases blood and renal cortical acid content in rats. Am J Physiol. 1998;274[Renal Physiol. 43]:F97–103.
12. Sun X, Yang LV, Tiegs BC, et al. Deletion of the pH sensor GPR4 decreases renal acid excretion. J Am Soc Nephrol. 2010;21:1745–55.
13. Swan RC, Pitts RF. Neutralization of infused acid by nephrectomized dogs. J Clin Invest. 1955;34:205–12.
14. Lemann J, Litzow JR, Lennon EJ, et al. Studies on the mechanism by which chronic metabolic acidosis augments urinary calcium excretion in man. J Clin Invest. 1967;46:1318–28.
15. Bushinsky DA. Net calcium efflux from live bone during chronic metabolic but not respiratory acidosis. Am J Physiol. 1989;256:F836–42.

Chapter 2
Metabolic Acidosis: Physiology, Presentation, and Diagnosis

Melvin E. Laski

Introduction

To diagnose metabolic acidosis the clinician must first prove the patient actually has acidosis. Patients with low serum bicarbonate (HCO_3) concentration, or hypobicarbonatemia, are commonly assumed to have metabolic acidosis, but hypobicarbonatemia is also an expected consequence of respiratory alkalosis (Fig. 2.1). In the absence of a simultaneous blood pH measurement a low serum HCO_3 concentration cannot distinguish which condition is present. This is particularly true when hypobicarbonatemia is found in an asymptomatic and stable patient. Addressing this challenge is aided by considering the patient's history. The determination of blood gas data in a patient with shock, known or suspected ingestion of toxin, or clinical diabetic ketoacidosis provides useful information, and in sepsis is a standard of care. A low arterial blood pH with hypobicarbonatemia indicates metabolic acidosis. If the blood pH is normal or high, hypobicarbonatemia is due to respiratory alkalosis or to multiple, concurrent (mixed), acid–base disorders.

Metabolic acidosis is a primary pathophysiological process characterized by hypobicarbonatemia resulting from either the loss of HCO_3 or the gain of non-volatile acid, the latter because of increased endogenous acid production above the kidney's normal acid excretory capacity or because of reduced kidney ability to excrete a patient's baseline load of endogenously produced acid. Hypobicarbonatemia develops because HCO_3 is lost from the body, most commonly by way of the urine or the gastrointestinal tract and is replaced by Cl^-, or alternatively, because HCO_3 is consumed in buffering non-volatile acid and is replaced by the anion of that acid. These two causalities are distinguished by calculation of the serum anion gap.

M.E. Laski, M.D. (✉)
Department of Internal Medicine, Texas Tech University Health Sciences Center,
3601 4th Street, Lubbock, TX 79430, USA
e-mail: Melvin.laski@ttuhsc.edu

© Springer Science+Business Media New York 2016
D.E. Wesson (ed.), *Metabolic Acidosis*, DOI 10.1007/978-1-4939-3463-8_2

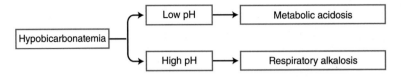

Fig. 2.1 Blood pH determines the meaning of hypobicarbonatemia (simple disorders)

The Use of the Serum Anion Gap [1, 2]

The serum anion gap is the arithmetical difference between the serum sodium concentration and the sum of the concentration of measured anions (HCO_3 and Cl^-). Thus:

$$\text{Anion gap}(AG) = [Na^+] - ([Cl^-] + [HCO_3]).$$

The normal anion gap (AG) is defined as 9 ± 3 meq/L, but might be as much as 12 ± 3 meq/L, depending on the local laboratory techniques for electrolyte measurement. Most of the "missing/unmeasured" anions are side chains of serum albumin. The serum albumin concentration therefore directly affects the gap. One anticipates a 2.5 meq/L decrease in anion gap for each 1 g/dL decrease in the serum albumin value below 4.5 [3]. Other proteins also contribute to the gap. Cationic side chains of immune globulins bind Cl^- and lower the AG. When immune globulins are increased, as occurs in multiple myeloma or in monoclonal gammopathy of unknown significance, the anion gap may become quite small.

The anion gap is relevant only when considering a patient with acidemia. Alkalemia exposes the anionic side chains of albumin and increases the anion gap. The anion gap might be particularly misleading during respiratory alkalosis, in which there are both low HCO_3 concentration and increased anion gap. Measuring blood pH eliminates misinterpretation.

The anion gap is used to limit the differential diagnosis of metabolic acidosis (Fig. 2.2). Normal anion gap metabolic acidosis, or hyperchloremic metabolic acidosis, results from (1) ingestion of hydrochloric acid, ammonium Cl^-, or arginine hydrochloride; (2) the inability to normally excrete metabolically produced acid in the urine due to distal renal tubular acidosis (RTA), advanced chronic kidney disease (CKD), or urinary diversion to the colon; or (3) the uncompensated loss of HCO_3 in proximal RTA, diarrhea, or pancreato-cutaneous fistula. In each instance the HCO_3 that is lost from the body or consumed by buffering is replaced by Cl^- and hyperchloremic metabolic acidosis results.

Normal AG metabolic acidosis or hyperchloremic metabolic acidosis		Anion gap metabolic acidosis		
Acid ingestion	Hydrochloric acid	Overproduction	Ketoacidosis	Diabetic ketoacidosis
	Ammonium chloride			Starvation ketoacidosis
	Arginine chloride		Lactic acidosis	Type A
Acid retention	Distal renal tubular acidosis			Type B
				D lactate
	Renal acidosis in CKD		Uremia	
	Ureteral diversion to colon	Ingestion	Ethylene glycol	
Bicarbonate loss	Proximal renal tubular acidosis		Methanol	
			Salicylate	
	Diarrhea		Paraldehyde	
	Pancreato-cutaneous fistula		Pyroglutamic acid	

Fig. 2.2 Serum anion gap in metabolic acidosis

Hyperchloremic Metabolic Acidosis [1, 2, 4, 5]

Mechanistically, the presence or absence of hyperchloremic metabolic acidosis is determined by the difference between the rate of addition of an acid with a non-Cl^- anion and the rate of excretion (by the kidney) of the accompanying non-Cl^- anion of the added acid with recovery of Cl^- to replace the excreted non-Cl^- anion, leading to secondary Cl^- retention [6]. Specifically, if the rate of excretion of the anion of the added non-Cl^- acid with secondary Cl^- retention is equal to the rate of addition of the non-Cl^--containing acid, hyperchloremic metabolic acidosis will result. If the rate of excretion of the non-Cl^- anion with secondary Cl^- retention is less than the rate of addition of the acid with the non-Cl^- anion, the patient will have an increased anion gap and therefore an anion gap metabolic acidosis.

The medical history nevertheless remains a critical part of patient evaluation and is most useful in diagnosing hyperchloremic metabolic acidosis due to diarrhea, pancreato-cutaneous fistula, amphotericin exposure, or urinary diversion. However, diarrhea in laxative abuse is often denied by patients. Hydrochloric acid or ammonium Cl^- ingestion is only seen in clinical research, but excessive arginine hydrochloride is sometimes present in total parenteral nutrition; review of the patient's chart should reveal this. Arginine HCl induced acidosis is far more likely in the setting of diminished GFR.

History is less useful in diagnosing RTA. Pure proximal RTA might cause poor growth in children, bone disease, and deafness. Renal rickets may be the presenting feature in the De Toni–Fanconi syndrome. Classic distal RTA may present with kidney stones and osteoporosis, and the effects of accompanying hypokalemia may be significant. Hyperkalemic distal RTA comes to clinical attention in most instances because of the associated hyperkalemia and less commonly because of the non-anion gap metabolic acidosis and can be caused by hyporeninism, hypoaldosteronism, and obstructive uropathy. The most common historical precedent for the latter is symptoms of prostatism.

In most circumstances of plasma acidemia (higher than normal $[H^+]$ which is equivalent to a lower than normal pH), the physiologically appropriate kidney response is to reduce urine pH below 5.5. In the setting of acidosis (net gain of H^+ in body fluids due to addition of H^+ or loss of HCO_3), the normal kidney also increases ammonium (NH_4^+) excretion, but urine NH_4^+ is rarely measured in clinical practice. Instead, clinicians more typically calculate the urine anion gap (UAG) as an indirect assessment of NH_4^+ from the concentration of other ions present in the urine [7].

$$\text{Urine anion gap (UAG)} = ([Na^+]_u + [K^+]_u) - [Cl^-]_u.$$

The HCO_3 concentration is insignificant in acid urine with $pH \le 6$ and is therefore disregarded. The UAG is measureable only when urine pH is low (≤ 6) because the concentration of bicarbonate may be significant in more alkaline urine. The UAG is best interpretable when Cl^- is the major urine anion.

The UAG is normally negative in acid urine because in the presence of high urine NH_4^+, NH_4^+ complexed with Cl^- makes the urine Cl^- concentration exceed the sum of the measured cations Na^+ and K^+. In this way, the UAG serves as a surrogate measure of urinary NH_4^+. The UAG should exceed -20 to -30 meq/L during metabolic acidosis. A patient with hyperchloremic metabolic acidosis and a urine pH over 5.5 or a positive UAG has RTA until proven otherwise. Several distinct types of RTA exist (Table 2.1).

When the urine pH exceeds 5.5 or the UAG is positive in the presence of metabolic acidosis the evaluation of RTA continues as shown in Fig. 2.3. Although classical distal RTA and proximal RTA are both characterized by hypokalemia and hyperchloremic metabolic acidosis, in classic distal RTA the urine pH typically exceeds 5.5 whereas the urine pH is typically <5.5 in untreated proximal RTA. This is because in proximal RTA distal nephron function is intact so the patient is able to lower urine pH appropriately when there is not excess HCO_3 delivery to the distal nephron. Proximal RTA without other disorders of proximal tubule function is rare. Proximal RTA is almost always part of generalized proximal tubule dysfunction as in the De Toni–Fanconi syndrome, which includes glycosuria during euglycemia, phosphaturia, uricosuria, and generalized aminoaciduria. To confirm proximal RTA is present the clinician infuses sodium HCO_3 to raise the blood HCO_3 over 18 meq/L which exceeds the ability of the defective proximal tubule to fully absorb in increased HCO_3, leading to excess HCO_3 delivered to the distal nephron. The clinician attempting to make the diagnosis of proximal RTA then measures the fractional excretion of HCO_3 ($FE_{HCO_3}\%$) where

$$FE_{HCO_3}\% = ([HCO_3]_u \times V) / [HCO_3]_p) / ([Cr]_u \times V) / [Cr]_p).$$

The $FE_{HCO_3}\%$ exceeds 10 % in proximal RTA when serum HCO_3 is >18 mmol/L.

Table 2.1 Renal tubular acidosis

	Defect	Clinical characteristics	Urine findings	Tests
Isolated proximal RTA (Type 2)	Depressed proximal tubule bicarbonate absorption	Bicarbonate <18 mmol/L, hypokalemia; carbonic anhydrase inhibitors	Urine pH normally <5.5 at baseline	$FE_{bicarbonate}$ % > 10 % if serum bicarbonate raised to 18 mmol/L by infusion
De Toni–Fanconi syndrome (Type 2)	Generalized proximal tubular dysfunction	Hypokalemia, hypouricemia, hypophosphatemia, bicarbonate <18 mmol/L, congenital syndromes, renal rickets	Baseline urine pH <5.5; glycosuria, phosphaturia, uricosuria, aminoaciduria	$FE_{bicarbonate}$ % > 10 % if serum bicarbonate raised to 18 mmol/L by infusion
Classic distal RTA (Type 1)	Impaired collecting duct proton secretion	Very low bicarbonate, hypokalemia, kidney stones, nephrocalcinosis	Urine pH>5.5 during acidemia	Urine pH
Hyperkalemic distal RTA (Type 4)	Mineralocorticoid deficiency or resistance; generalized failure of distal nephron ion transport	Bicarbonate 15–22, potassium >5.5; seen in urinary tract obstruction, interstitial renal disease, adrenal disorders	Positive UAG may be present; urine pH may be >5.5 or normal	Urine pH, UAG
Backleak RTA	Backleak of acid due to amphotericin	Hypokalemia; exposure to amphotericin	Urine pH>5.5, urinary K wasting	Urine pH; difference between urine and blood PCO_2 during bicarbonate and phosphate infusion is normal
CKD	Inadequate ammonium excretion	Low GFR	Urine pH<5.5, low UAG	Urine pH; UAG, eGFR

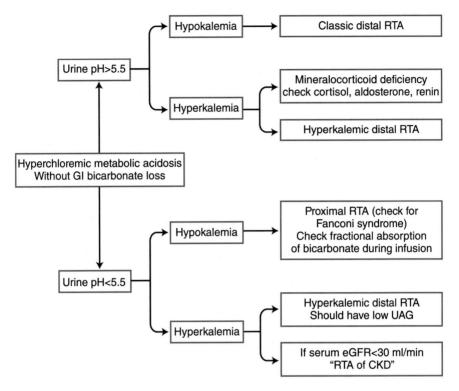

Fig. 2.3 Diagnosis of RTA by urine pH, urine anion gap, and serum potassium

Amphotericin causes hyperchloremic metabolic acidosis with hypokalemia and urine pH > 5.5. Amphotericin introduces a molecular channel through which potassium (K^+) leaks out from the renal tubular cell to the urine and protons backleak from the urine to the cell. As a result the kidney cannot maintain a low urine pH even though protons (H^+) are secreted normally, and K^+ is lost in the urine. Similarly, when ureters are diverted to the colon there is acid backleak and loss of K^+ Cl^- in stool.

Hyperkalemia and hyperchloremic metabolic acidosis characterize Type 4 (hyperkalemic) distal RTA. If the urine pH is < 5.5 UAG will be positive due to impaired renal NH_4^+ excretion. Blood tests can then dissect whether the problem is adrenal failure (low cortisol and low aldosterone), isolated aldosterone deficiency (low aldosterone but normal or high renin), or the most common cause of Type 4 distal RTA, hyporeninemic hypoaldosteronism (low renin, low aldosterone). Hyperkalemic distal RTA due to tubule cell injury in urinary tract obstruction or interstitial renal disease may have urine pH > 5.5. Medications may cause hyperkalemic distal RTA. Drugs designed to block the response to aldosterone are easily understood as potential causes, but trimethoprim (most often ingested in combination with sulfamethoxazole), and pentamidine are now commonly seen to cause hyperkalemia and potentially can cause hyperchloremic acidosis. This should be considered in the context of care of a patient with HIV infection.

Metabolic Acidosis with Increased Anion Gap [1, 2, 4, 8]

Overproduction Acidosis

Anion gap metabolic acidosis is easier to diagnose than non-anion gap or hyperchloremic metabolic acidosis. The patient with diabetic ketoacidosis is usually hyperglycemic and often has a well-established history of type 1 DM. Volume depletion is almost invariably present and is due to the combination of glycosuria-induced osmotic diuresis with loss of $H_2O + NaCl$ and poor NaCl intake due to GI upset, the latter often accompanied with vomiting and further NaCl loss. The lack of insulin allows for excess glucose release to the serum but the extremely high blood glucose levels in diabetic ketoacidosis are facilitated by volume depletion-induced decreased kidney filtration that subsequently limits further glucose loss in the urine. Respiratory response to the metabolic acidosis (increased ventilation with decreased PCO_2) is marked, and Kussmaul respiration is classic. Starvation ketoacidosis is harder to recognize than diabetic ketoacidosis because it is less severe and because the routine use of glucose-containing intravenous fluids often inadvertently treats starvation ketosis in this setting of anion gap metabolic acidosis. Clinicians might find it difficult to distinguish starvation ketoacidosis from other forms of anion gap metabolic acidosis not associated with ketone bodies because of the particular ketone bodies often associated with starvation ketosis. The key diagnostic test is the detection of ketone bodies in the blood or urine but there is one caveat. The nitroprusside moiety in the common test for ketone bodies detects only the oxidized ketones (acetone). In some patients, particularly alcoholics, "reduced" ketones (β-hydroxybutyrate) predominate and so their anion gap metabolic acidosis might be associated with a "negative" test for ketone bodies. As β-hydroxybutyrate measurement is not commonly available one often proceeds with treatment for ketoacidosis with some uncertainty. Diabetic ketoacidosis is treated with insulin to suppress glucagon and drive glucose into insulin sensitive cells. Starvation ketoacidosis responds to provision of carbohydrates.

Lactic acidosis should never be missed. The arterial lactate level should be measured routinely in patients with anion gap metabolic acidosis, because lactic acidosis may be concurrent in every other form of anion gap acidosis. Carbohydrate metabolism can be compartmentalized into a cytoplasmic or anaerobic phase characterized by glycolysis, and a mitochondrial, aerobic phase that is characterized by the Krebs cycle. Glycolysis produces lactate, pyruvate, and ATP; the Krebs cycle oxidizes pyruvate to carbon dioxide and water and produces ATP and NADH. NADH is needed to convert lactate to pyruvate. Lactic acidosis develops when mitochondrial (aerobic) metabolism fails due to an insufficient oxygen supply or tissue hypoxia (Type A), or to disturbances in the machinery of aerobic metabolism that might be caused by advanced liver disease, inborn errors of metabolism, or poisoning (Type B). In the absence of NADH from oxidative metabolism the lactic acid generated by glycolysis accumulates. When a patient presents to the hospital in shock, lactic acidosis should be actively sought, both on arrival and whenever the patient's condition worsens significantly. The inborn errors of metabolism associated with lactic acidosis present in complex ways which are characteristic of the particular genetic syndrome involved.

D-Lactic acid is a product of certain gut bacteria which are normally present in small amounts so its typically small amount of production is usually of no clinical consequence. Nevertheless, when these bacteria grow to become a greater proportion of gut bacteria as might occur in patients with previous surgery that created an intestinal blind loop where bacterial overgrowth occurs and these bacteria receive large quantities of carbohydrate, D-lactic acidosis can occur. Patients with D-lactic acidosis have altered mental status and unexplained anion gap acidosis. Lactate levels are reported as normal because standard laboratory tests for lactate detect only L-lactate. If clinicians suspect D-lactic acidosis, they must specifically request this test. Treatment is to alter the diet to reduce carbohydrate delivery to these gut bacteria and to reduce bacterial overgrowth.

Anion Gap Acidosis Due to Acid Ingestion or Retention

Methanol ingestion is often inadvertent. The most common scenario is the intake of homemade drink by alcoholics or inmates in prison settings. Any available solvent may be added in this situation. Alcoholics may also drink Sterno® filtered through bread or other material that they believe, incorrectly, removes the toxic qualities. One ounce of methanol ingested can kill; a mole of methanol fits in a shot glass. Ingestion of methanol produces intoxication, "snowy vision" and blindness, formication, coma, and death. There is not only anion gap metabolic acidosis but also severe disagreement between measured and calculated serum osmolarity—the osmolar gap.

Calculated serum osmolarity = $([Na^+]_p \times 2) + (BUN / 2.8) + ([glucose]_p / 18)$;

Osmolar gap = measured osmolarity − calculated osmolarity

The calculated osmolarity normally provides an estimate within 10 mOsm of the measured value. In methanol, ethylene glycol, and paraldehyde ingestion the osmolar gap exceeds 15 mOsm. Methanol metabolism by alcohol dehydrogenase generates formic acid and formaldehyde, which are highly toxic. The appropriate treatment is general patient support, the inhibition of alcohol dehydrogenase by fomepizole or ethanol infusion, and hemodialysis. Treatment is emergent when ingestion is suspected.

Ethylene glycol is a sweet tasting intoxicant. Its ingestion has become rare due to its omission from new, non-toxic automotive antifreeze, and it is easier to diagnose since fluorescein has been added to antifreeze. Exposing the urine to a Wood's light detects fluorescence. Ethylene glycol ingestion increases the osmolar gap. Ethylene glycol metabolites glycolic acid and oxalic acid do the greatest harm. Oxalic acid causes kidney failure and glycolic acid causes lactic acidosis. The treatment is general patient support, infusion of fomepizole or ethanol to inhibit alcohol dehydrogenase, and hemodialysis to remove the toxins.

Paraldehyde ingestion is no longer a clinically relevant because this small molecule sedative/hypnotic is no longer used. The keys to its diagnosis were its unique odor and an increased osmolar gap.

Salicylate overdose causes two acid–base disorders, respiratory alkalosis due to stimulation of the respiratory center, and AG metabolic acidosis caused by two mechanisms: accumulation of salicylate anions, and lactic acidosis due to inhibition of oxidative phosphorylation. Salicylate levels are readily obtained. Treatment includes support, urine alkalization to increase salicylate excretion, and hemodialysis.

Anion gap positive metabolic acidosis associated with acetaminophen has been described in critically ill patients [9]. The major acid anion proved to be pyroglutamic acid generated in the synthesis of glutathione. Acetaminophen induced depletion of glutathione leads to increased glutathione synthesis and raises pyroglutamic acid production. The condition is rare compared to the use of the drug and might involve an underlying abnormality of glutathione metabolism.

Anion gap metabolic acidosis is also caused by severely decreased glomerular filtration rate (GFR) that, among many adverse consequences of this state of disordered metabolism known as uremia [10], leads to failure to excrete ingested and metabolically produced acid. Uremic acidosis develops in the context of advanced renal failure, either chronic or acute. Anion gap acidosis in these patients is due to the retention of acidic uremic waste products. Only a minority of patients have pure anion gap metabolic acidosis due to uremia. Most such patients exhibit a mix of "gap" acidosis and hyperchloremic acidosis due to RTA or the failure to adequately produce ammonium Cl^-. A few patients have pure hyperchloremic acidosis. Mild metabolic acidosis is probably present in most untreated patients with eGFR under 30 ml/min/1.73 m^2 and its presence or absence is due in part to their dietary acid content [11]. That is, the higher the dietary content of fixed acid in a patient with compromised ability to excrete metabolically produced acid, the more likely the patient is to exhibit metabolic acidosis. Treatment of mild to moderate uremic acidosis and acidosis of CKD is clinically beneficial and too often ignored.

A final issue to consider is the assessment and diagnosis of patients with metabolic acidosis who have multiple acid–base disorders [4]. If a patient with metabolic acidosis has a decline in HCO_3 concentration from 25 (ΔHCO_3) that exceeds the increase in the serum anion gap (ΔAG) by more than 20 %, superimposed hyperchloremic metabolic acidosis may be present. If the ΔHCO_3 is more than 20 % less than the ΔAG, the patient may have metabolic alkalosis in addition to metabolic acidosis. Physiologic respiratory response with decreased PCO_2 is expected in metabolic acidosis but this is not to be confused with simultaneous respiratory alkalosis. The PCO_2 should decrease by 1.2 mm/Hg for each 1 meq/L fall in HCO_3, and the pH will increase toward but will not become normal. If the fall in PCO_2 exceeds the expected amount the patient has respiratory alkalosis in addition to metabolic acidosis. If the PCO_2 fails to decrease as predicted, respiratory acidosis is likely superimposed.

References

1. Toto RD, Alpern RJ. Metabolic acid–base disorders. In: Kokko JP, Tannen RL, editors. Fluids and electrolytes. 3rd ed. Philadelphia: WB Saunders; 1996. p. 201–66.
2. DuBose Jr TD. Disorders of acid–base balance. In: Brenner BM, editor. Brenner & Rector's the kidney. 8th ed. Philadelphia: WD Saunders; 2008. p. 505–46.
3. Feldman M, Soni N, Dickson B. Influence of hypoalbuminemia or hyperalbuminemia on the serum anion gap. J Lab Clin Med. 2005;146:317–20.
4. Emmett M. Diagnosis of simple and mixed disorders. In: DuBose TD, Hamm LL, editors. Acid–base and electrolyte disorders: a companion to Brenner and Rector's the kidney. Philadelphia: WD Saunders; 2002. p. 41–54.
5. Laski ME, Kaldas A. Renal tubular acidosis. In Best Practice, BMJ. 2013. https://online.epocrates.com/u/2911239/Renal+tubular+acidosis.
6. Krapf R, Alpern RJ, Seldin DW. Clinical syndromes of metabolic acidosis. In: Seldin DW, Giebisch G, editors. The kidney. Philadelphia: Lippincott Williams & Wilkins; 2000. p. 2055–72.
7. Laski ME, Kurtzman NA. Evaluation of acid–base disorders from the urine. In: Seldin DW, Giebisch G, editors. The regulation of acid–base balance. New York, NY: Raven; 1989. p. 265–83.
8. Laski ME, Wesson DE. Lactic acidosis. In: DuBose TD, Hamm LL, editors. Acid–base and electrolyte disorders: a companion to Brenner and Rector's the kidney. Philadelphia: WD Saunders; 2002. p. 68–83.
9. Mizock BA, Belyaev S, Mecher C. Unexplained metabolic acidosis in critically ill patients: the role of pyroglutamic acid. Intensive Care Med. 2004;30:502–5.
10. Kraut JA, Kurtz I. Metabolic acidosis of CKD: diagnosis, clinical characteristics, and treatment. Am J Kidney Dis. 2005;45:978–93.
11. Adeva MM, Souto G. Diet-induced metabolic acidosis. Clin Nutr. 2011;30:416–21.

Chapter 3
Etiologic Causes of Metabolic Acidosis I: The High Anion Gap Acidoses

Thomas D. DuBose Jr.

High Anion Gap Acidoses

The anion gap (AG) should always be corrected for the prevailing albumin concentration (for each g/dL decrease in albumin below the normal value of 4 g/dL, add 2.5 mEq/L to the traditionally calculated AG to obtain the corrected AG). A normal AG in patients with a normal serum albumin concentration and otherwise normal metabolic status is 10 ± 2 mEq/L. Corrected AG values above 10 ± 2 mEq/L represent a high AG metabolic acidosis. When corrected in this manner, the anion gap [1] serves a useful tool in the initial differentiation of the types of metabolic acidoses and should always be considered as an important component of understanding the pathophysiology of the specific defect. A high AG acidosis denotes addition of an acid other than hydrochloric acid or its equivalent to the ECF and is caused by the accumulation of organic acids. This may occur if the anion does not undergo glomerular filtration (e.g., uremic acid anions), or if, because of alteration in metabolic pathways (ketoacidosis, L-lactic acidosis), the anion cannot be utilized immediately. Theoretically, with a pure AG acidosis, the increment in the AG above the normal value of 10 ± 3 mEq/L (ΔAG), should equal the decrease in bicarbonate concentration below the normal value of 25 mEq/L (ΔHCO_3^-). When this relationship is considered, circumstances in which the increment in the AG exceeds the decrement in bicarbonate ($\Delta AG > \Delta HCO_3^-$) suggest the coexistence of a metabolic alkalosis. By contrast, circumstances in which the increment in the AG is less than the decrement in bicarbonate ($\Delta AG < \Delta HCO_3^-$) suggest the coexistence of a non-AG metabolic acidosis.

Common causes of a high gap acidosis include (1) lactic acidosis, (2) ketoacidosis, (3) toxin- or poison-induced acidosis, and (4) uremic acidosis. Clinical examples are summarized in Table 3.1.

T.D. DuBose Jr., M.D., M.A.C.P., F.A.S.N. (✉)
Section on General Internal Medicine, Wake Forest School of Medicine,
Medical Center Boulevard, Winston Salem, NC 27157, USA
e-mail: tdubose@wakehealth.edu

© Springer Science+Business Media New York 2016
D.E. Wesson (ed.), *Metabolic Acidosis*, DOI 10.1007/978-1-4939-3463-8_3

Table 3.1 Causes of high anion gap metabolic acidosis

Lactic acidosis	Toxins
Ketoacidosis	Ethylene glycol
Diabetic	Methanol
Alcoholic	Salicylates
Starvation	Propylene glycol
	Pyroglutamic acid
	Kidney failure (acute and chronic)

Lactic Acidosis

Pathophysiology

Lactic acid can exist in two forms: L (levorotatory)-lactic acid and D (dextrorotatory)-lactic acid. In mammals, only the levorotatory form is a product of mammalian metabolism. D-Lactate can accumulate in humans only as a by-product of metabolism of carbohydrate by bacteria which abnormally accumulate and overgrow in the gastrointestinal tract as might occur with a "blind loop" in bowel, with jejunal bypass, or short bowel syndrome. L-Lactic acidosis is one of the most common forms of a high AG acidosis, and hospital chemical laboratories routinely measure L-lactic acid levels, not D-lactic acid levels. Consequently, the clinician who suspects D-lactic acidosis must ask the clinical laboratory to specifically measure D-lactic acid.

Lactic acid metabolism, although similar to that of pyruvate, is in a metabolic cul-de-sac with pyruvate as its only outlet [2]. In most cells, the major metabolic pathway for pyruvate is oxidation in the mitochondria to acetyl–coenzyme A by the enzyme pyruvate dehydrogenase within the mitochondria. The overall reaction may be expressed as in Eq. (3.1):

$$\text{Pyruvate}^- + \text{NADH} \Leftrightarrow \text{lactate}^- + \text{NAD} + \text{H}^+ \qquad (3.1)$$

Normally, this cytosolic reaction catalyzed by the enzyme lactate dehydrogenase (LDH) is close to equilibrium, so that the law of mass action applies and the equation is rearranged as (3.2):

$$[\text{Lactate}^-] = K_{eq}[\text{H}^+]\frac{\text{NADH}}{\text{NAD}^+} \qquad (3.2)$$

The concentration of lactate is a function of the equilibrium constant (K_{eq}), the pyruvate concentration, the cytosolic pH, and the intracellular redox state represented by the concentration ratio of reduced to oxidized nicotinamide adenine dinucleotide or [NADH]/[NAD$^+$] [2].

Because K_{eq} and intracellular H$^+$ concentration are relatively constant, the normal lactate/pyruvate concentration ratio (1.0/0.1 mEq/L) is proportional to the

NADH/NAD$^+$ concentration ratio. Therefore the lactate/pyruvate ratio and the ratio of reduced to the oxidized forms of these molecules is a function of the cellular redox potential (3.3):

$$\frac{[NADH]}{[NAD^+]^+} \propto \frac{[Lactate]}{[Pyruvate]} \propto \frac{[\beta\ hydroxybutyrate]}{[acetoacetate]} \propto \frac{[ethanol]}{acetaldehyde} \tag{3.3}$$

If the lactate concentration is high compared with that of pyruvate, NAD$^+$ will be depleted, and the NADH/NAD$^+$ ratio will increase. The production of lactic acid has been estimated to be about 15–20 mEq/kg/day in normal humans [3], but can be increased by ischemia, seizures, extreme exercise, leukemia, and alkalosis [2]. The increase in production occurs principally through enhanced phosphofructokinase activity.

Decreased lactate consumption may also lead to L-lactic acidosis. The principal organs for lactate removal include the liver, kidneys, and skeletal muscle [4]. Hepatic utilization of lactate can be impeded by: poor perfusion of the liver; defective active transport of lactate into cells; and inadequate metabolic conversion of lactate into pyruvate because of altered intracellular pH, redox state, or enzyme activity. Examples of states causing impaired hepatic lactate removal include primary diseases of the liver, enzymatic defects, tissue anoxia or ischemia, severe acidosis, and altered redox states, as occurs with alcohol intoxication, fructose consumption by fructose-intolerant individuals, or administration of nucleoside reverse transcriptase inhibitors [2, 5, 6] or biguanides such as metformin [2, 7, 8]. Since thiamine is a cofactor for pyruvate dehydrogenase that catalyzes the oxidative decarboxylation of pyruvate to acetyl–coenzyme A under aerobic conditions, it is not surprising that deaths have been reported due to refractory lactic acidosis secondary to thiamine deficiency [9]. When pyruvate cannot be metabolized with thiamine deficiency, excess pyruvate is converted to hydrogen ions and lactate.

Pathogenesis and Clinical Spectrum

According to the historical classification of the L-lactic acidoses, type A L-lactic acidosis is due to tissue hypoperfusion or acute hypoxia, whereas type B L-lactic acidosis is associated with common diseases, drugs and toxins, and hereditary and miscellaneous disorders [2]. Lactate concentrations are mildly increased in various nonpathologic states (e.g., exercise), but the magnitude of the elevation is generally small. A lactate concentration greater than 4 mmol/L (normal is 0.67–1.8 mmol/L) is taken as evidence that the metabolic acidosis is the result of lactic-acid acidosis.

Tissue underperfusion and acute underoxygenation at the tissue level (tissue hypoxia) are the most common causes of type A lactic acidosis. Inadequate cardiac output, of either the low-output or the high-output variety, is the most frequent cause, but severe arterial hypoxemia can also generate L-lactic acidosis. The prognosis is related to the increment in plasma L-lactate and the severity of the acidemia [2, 8, 10].

A number of medical disorders (without tissue hypoxia) may cause type B L-lactic acidosis. Hepatic failure reduces hepatic lactate metabolism, and leukemia increases lactate production. Severe anemia, especially as a result of iron deficiency or methemoglobulinemia, may cause lactic acidosis. Among patients in the critical care unit the most common cause of L-lactic acidosis is bowel ischemia and infarction. Malignant cells produce more lactate than normal cells even under aerobic conditions. This phenomenon is magnified if the tumor expands rapidly and outstrips its blood supply. Therefore, exceptionally large tumors may be associated with severe L-lactic acidosis. Seizures, extreme exertion, heat stroke, and tumor lysis syndrome may all cause L-lactic acidosis.

Several drugs and toxins predispose to L-lactic acidosis. Of these, metformin is the most widely reported to have this effect [2, 7, 8], but metformin-induced lactic acidosis is at higher risk in patients with chronic kidney disease (and is contraindicated when the serum creatinine exceeds 1.4 mg/dL), or whenever there is hypoperfusion or hypotension, including severe volume depletion (especially in the elderly), shock, septicemia, CHF, or a recent AMI.

In patients with HIV infection, nucleoside analogs predispose to toxic effects on mitochondria by inhibiting DNA polymerase-γ. Therefore, hyperlactatemia is common with anti-HIV therapy, but the serum L-lactate level is usually only mildly elevated [2, 5, 6, 11]. However, with severe concurrent illness pronounced lactic acidosis may occur in association with hepatic steatosis [2, 6] and a high mortality.

Translational Approach

The overall mortality of patients with L-lactic acidosis is approximately 60 %, but approaches 100 % in those with coexisting hypotension or multiorgan dysfunction [2]. The only effective form of therapy for L-lactic acidosis is to correct the underlying condition initiating the disruption in normal lactate metabolism. Cessation of acid production by improvement of tissue oxygenation, restoration of the circulating fluid volume, improvement or augmentation of cardiac function, resection of ischemic tissue, and antibiotics is necessary for type A L-lactic acidosis.

Alkali therapy is generally advocated for acute, severe acidemia (pH of <7.0) to improve myocardial inotropy and lactate utilization. However, $NaHCO_3$ therapy in large amounts can depress cardiac performance and exacerbate the acidemia. Paradoxically, bicarbonate therapy activates phosphofructokinase, which is regulated by intracellular pH, thereby increasing lactate production. For all of these reasons, $NaHCO_3$ should be used cautiously with the goal of increasing the plasma $[HCO_3^-]$ to no more than 5–8 mmol/L.

If the underlying cause of the L-lactic acidosis can be remedied, blood lactate will be reconverted to HCO_3^-. The bicarbonate derived metabolically from lactate conversion is additive to any new HCO_3^- generated by kidney mechanisms during acidosis and from exogenous alkali therapy might lead to an "overshoot" alkalosis.

D-*Lactic Acidosis*

The typical manifestations of D-lactate acidosis are episodic encephalopathy and high AG acidosis in association with short bowel syndrome. D-Lactic acidosis has been described in patients with bowel obstruction, jejunal bypass, short bowel, or ischemic bowel disease. Ileus or stasis is associated with overgrowth of flora in the gastrointestinal tract, which is exacerbated by a high-carbohydrate diet [2]. D-Lactate acidosis occurs when fermentation by colonic bacteria in the intestine causes D-lactate to accumulate so that it can be absorbed into the circulation. Serum D-lactate levels of greater than 3 mmol/L confirm the diagnosis. Treatment with a low-carbohydrate diet and antibiotics (neomycin, vancomycin, or metronidazole) is often effective [12–15].

Ketoacidosis

Diabetic Ketoacidosis

Diabetic ketoacidosis (DKA) is due to increased fatty acid metabolism and accumulation of ketoacids (acetoacetate and β-hydroxybutyrate) as a result of insulin deficiency or resistance and elevated glucagon levels. DKA is usually seen in insulin-dependent diabetes mellitus upon cessation of insulin therapy or during an illness, such as an infection, gastroenteritis, pancreatitis, or myocardial infarction, which increases insulin requirements acutely. The accumulation of ketoacids accounts for the increment in the AG, which is accompanied, most often, by hyperglycemia (glucose level of >300 mg/dL) [15–17].

Alcoholic Ketoacidosis

Some patients with chronic alcoholism, especially binge drinkers, who discontinue food intake while continuing alcohol consumption, may develop the alcoholic form of ketoacidosis [12, 13, 18]. Often the onset of vomiting and abdominal pain with volume depletion leads to cessation of alcohol consumption [16, 17]. The metabolic acidosis may be severe but is accompanied by only modestly deranged glucose levels, which are usually low but may be slightly elevated [15, 18]. The net result of the deranged metabolic state is ketosis. The acidosis is primarily due to elevated levels of ketones, which exist predominantly in the form of β-hydroxybutyrate because of the altered redox state induced by the metabolism of alcohol. Compared with patients with DKA, patients with AKA have lower plasma glucose concentrations and higher β-hydroxybutyrate/acetoacetate and lactate/pyruvate ratios [16, 17]. Because the standard clinical tests for ketone bodies do not detect the reduced ketoacid β-hydroxybutyrate, AKA patients with severe ketoacidosis comprised mostly of β-hydroxybutyrate might escape detection in the setting of a negative test for ketones if the clinician does not have a high index of suspicion. The typical high AG acidosis is often mixed with metabolic alkalosis (vomiting), respiratory alkalosis (alcoholic liver disease), lactic acidosis (hypoperfusion), and/or hyperchloremic acidosis (kidney excretion of ketoacids). Finally, elevation in the osmolar gap is usually accounted for by an increased blood alcohol level, but the differential diagnosis should always include ethylene glycol and/or methanol intoxication [16, 17].

Drug- and Toxin-Induced Acidosis

Salicylate

Intoxication with salicylates, although more common in children than in adults, may result in the development of a high AG metabolic acidosis, but [15] adult patients with salicylate intoxication usually have pure respiratory alkalosis or mixed respiratory alkalosis–metabolic acidosis [15]. A portion of the increase in the AG is due to the increase in plasma salicylate concentration, and the remainder is due to high ketone concentrations, present in as many as 40 % of adult salicylate-intoxicated patients in combination with increased L-lactic acid production, due to a direct drug effect and the result of the salicylate-induced decrease in PCO_2 [15, 19].

The Osmolar Gap and Toxin-Induced Metabolic Acidosis

Under most physiologic conditions, Na^+, urea, and glucose generate the osmotic pressure of blood. Serum osmolality is calculated according to the following expression (3.4):

$$Osmolality = 2[Na^+] + \frac{[BUN]}{2.8} + \frac{[Glucose(mg/dL)]}{18} \qquad (3.4)$$

The calculated and determined osmolality should agree within 10 mOsm/kg. When the measured osmolality exceeds the calculated osmolality by more than 10 mOsm/kg, one of two circumstances prevails. First, the serum Na^+ may be spuriously low, as occurs with hyperlipidemia or hyperproteinemia (pseudohyponatremia). Second, osmolytes other than sodium salts, glucose, or urea may have accumulated in plasma. Examples are infused mannitol, radiocontrast media, or other solutes, including the alcohols, ethylene glycol, and acetone, which can increase the osmolality in plasma. For these examples, the difference between the osmolality calculated from Eq. (3.4) and the measured osmolality is proportional to the concentration of the unmeasured solute. This difference, is known as the *osmo-*

lar gap, and becomes a very reliable and helpful screening tool in assessing for toxin-associated high AG acidosis.

Ethylene Glycol

Ingestion of ethylene glycol (EG), used in antifreeze, leads to a high AG metabolic [15, 20, 21] acidosis in addition to severe central nervous system, cardiopulmonary, and kidney damage. Disparity between the measured and calculated blood osmolality (high osmolar gap) is usually noted, especially in the first few hours after ingestion. Typically over time, as the EG is metabolized, the osmolar gap begins to fall and the anion gap begins to rise so that in advanced EG intoxication, the AG will be very high but the osmolar gap will narrow. The high AG is attributable to ethylene glycol metabolites, especially oxalic acid, glycolic acid, and other incompletely identified organic acids [21]. L-Lactic acid production also increases as a result of a toxic depression in the reaction rates of the citric acid cycle and altered intracellular redox state [21].

Methanol

Methanol has wide application in commercially available solvents and is used for industrial and automotive purposes. Sources include windshield wiper fluid, paint remover or thinner, deicing fluid, canned heating sources, varnish, and shellac. Ingestion of methanol (wood alcohol) causes metabolic acidosis in addition to severe optic nerve and central nervous system manifestations resulting from its metabolism to formic acid from formaldehyde [15, 20]. Lactic acids and ketoacids as well as other unidentified organic acids may contribute to the acidosis. Because of the low molecular mass of methanol (32 Da), an osmolar gap is usually present early in the course but declines as the anion gap increases, the latter reflecting the metabolism of methanol. Therapy for both methanol and ethylene glycol intoxication includes general supportive measures, fomepizole administration, and hemodialysis [22].

Pyroglutamic Acid

Pyroglutamic acid, or 5-oxoproline, is an intermediate in the γ-glutamyl cycle for the synthesis of glutathione. Acetaminophen ingestion can in rare cases deplete glutathione, which results in increased formation of γ-glutamyl cysteine, which is metabolized to pyroglutamic acid [23]. Accumulation of this intermediate has been reported in critically ill patients taking acetaminophen, usually with sepsis. Such patients have severe high AG acidosis and alterations in mental status [23].

Propylene Glycol

Propylene glycol is used as a vehicle for intravenous medications and some cosmetics and is metabolized to lactic acid by hepatic alcohol dehydrogenase. Numerous intravenous preparations contain propylene glycol as the vehicle (lorazepam, diazepam, pentobarbital, phenytoin, nitroglycerin, and TMP-SMX), and may accumulate and cause a high AG, high osmolar gap acidosis in patients receiving continuous infusion or higher dosages of these agents, especially in the presence of chronic kidney disease, chronic liver disease, alcohol abuse, or pregnancy [24, 25]. The acidosis is the result of accumulation of L-lactic acid, D-lactic acid, and L-acetaldehyde, but typically abates with cessation of the offending agent [26].

Uremia

Advanced chronic kidney disease eventually converts the non-gap metabolic acidosis of Stage 3–4 CKD to the typical high AG acidosis, or "uremic acidosis" of Stage 5 CKD [27]. Poor filtration plus continued reabsorption of poorly identified uremic organic anions contributes to the pathogenesis of this metabolic disturbance.

Classical uremic acidosis is characterized by a reduced rate of NH_4^+ production and excretion because of cumulative and significant loss of kidney mass [27–29]. Usually, acidosis does not occur until a major portion of the total functional nephron population has been compromised, because of the adaptation by surviving nephrons to increase ammoniagenesis.

Pathophysiological Basis of Correction of Acidosis of Chronic Kidney Failure

The uremic acidosis of advanced CKD requires oral alkali replacement to maintain the HCO_3^- concentration above 22 mEq/L. This can be accomplished with relatively modest amounts of alkali (1.0–1.5 mEq/kg/day of $NaHCO_3$ tablets). Alkali replacement serves to prevent the harmful effects of prolonged positive H^+ balance, especially progressive catabolism of muscle and loss of bone.

References

1. Emmet M. Diagnosis of simple and mixed disorders. In: DuBose TD, Hamm LL, editors. Acid–base and electrolyte disorders: a companion to Brenner and Rector's the kidney. Philadelphia: Saunders; 2002. p. 41–54.
2. Laski ME, Wesson DE. Lactic acidosis. In: DuBose TD, Hamm LL, editors. Acid–base and electrolyte disorders: a companion to Brenner and Rector's the kidney. Philadelphia: Saunders; 2002. p. 68–83.

3. DuBose TD, McDonald GA. Renal tubular acidosis. In: DuBose TD, Hamm LL, editors. Acid–base and electrolyte disorders: a companion to Brenner and Rector's the kidney. Philadelphia: Saunders; 2002. p. 189–206.
4. Goraya N, Simoni J, Jo CH, Wesson DE. A comparison of treating metabolic acidosis in CKD stage 4 hypertensive kidney disease with fruits and vegetables or sodium bicarbonate. Clin J Am Soc Nephrol. 2013;8:371–81.
5. John M, Mallal S. Hyperlactatemia syndromes in people with HIV infection. Curr Opin Infect Dis. 2002;15:23–9.
6. Cote HC, Brumme ZL, Craib KJ, et al. Changes in mitochondrial DNA as a marker of nucleoside toxicity in HIV-infected patients. N Engl J Med. 2002;346:811–20.
7. Lalau JD, Race JM. Lactic acidosis in metformin therapy. Drugs. 1999;58 Suppl 1:55–60.
8. Calabrese AT, Coley KC, DaPos SV, et al. Evaluation of prescribing practices: risk of lactic acidosis with metformin therapy. Arch Intern Med. 2002;162:434–7.
9. Romanski SA, McMahon MM. Metabolic acidosis and thiamine deficiency. Mayo Clin Proc. 1999;74:259–63.
10. Luft FC. Lactic acidosis update for critical care clinicians. J Am Soc Nephrol. 2001;12 Suppl 17:S15–9.
11. Gerard Y, Maulin L, Yazdanpanah Y, et al. Symptomatic hyperlactataemia: an emerging complication of antiretroviral therapy. AIDS. 2000;14:2723–30.
12. Uchida H, Yamamoto H, Kisaki Y, et al. D-Lactic acidosis in short-bowel syndrome managed with antibiotics and probiotics. J Pediatr Surg. 2004;39:634–6.
13. Jorens PG, Demey HE, Schepens PJ, et al. Unusual D-lactic acid acidosis from propylene glycol metabolism in overdose. J Toxicol Clin Toxicol. 2004;42:163–9.
14. Lalive PH, Hadengue A, Mensi N, Burkhard PR. Recurrent encephalopathy after small bowel resection. Implication of D-lactate. Rev Neurol (Paris). 2001;157:679–81.
15. Whitney GM, Szerlip HM. Acid–base disorders in the critical care setting. In: DuBose TD, Hamm LL, editors. Acid–base and electrolyte disorders: a companion to Brenner and Rector's the kidney. Philadelphia: Saunders; 2002. p. 165–87.
16. Halperin ML, Kamel KS, Cherney DZ. Ketoacidosis. In: DuBose TD, Hamm LL, editors. Acid–base and electrolyte disorders: a companion to Brenner and Rector's the kidney. Philadelphia: Saunders; 2002. p. 67–82.
17. Umpierrez GE, DiGirolamo M, Tuvlin JA, et al. Differences in metabolic and hormonal milieu in diabetic- and alcohol-induced ketoacidosis. J Crit Care. 2000;15:52–9.
18. DuBose TD, Alpern RJ. Renal tubular acidosis. In: The metabolic and molecular bases of inherited disease. New York: McGraw-Hill; 2001. p. 4983–5021.
19. Proudfoot AT, Krenzelok EP, Brent J, Vale JA. Does urine alkalinization increase salicylate elimination? If so, why? Toxicol Rev. 2003;22:129–36.
20. Brent J. Fomepizole for ethylene glycol and methanol poisoning. N Engl J Med. 2009;360:2216–23.
21. Fraser AD. Clinical toxicologic implications of ethylene glycol and glycolic acid poisoning. Ther Drug Monit. 2002;24:232–8.
22. Velez LI, Shepherd G, Lee YC, Keyes DC. Ethylene glycol ingestion treated only with fomepizole. J Med Toxicol. 2007;3:125–8.
23. Mizock BA, Belyaev S, Mecher C. Unexplained metabolic acidosis in critically ill patients: the role of pyroglutamic acid. Intensive Care Med. 2004;30:502–5.
24. Wilson KC, Reardon C, Farber HW. Propylene glycol toxicity in a patient receiving intravenous diazepam. N Engl J Med. 2000;343:815.
25. Zar T, Yusufzai I, Sullivan A, Graeber C. Acute kidney injury, hyperosmolality and metabolic acidosis associated with lorazepam. Nat Clin Pract Nephrol. 2007;3:515–20.
26. Loniewski I, Wesson DE. Bicarbonate therapy for prevention of chronic kidney disease progression. Kidney Int. 2014;85:529–35.
27. Kraut JA, Kurtz I. Metabolic acidosis of CKD: diagnosis, clinical characteristics, and treatment. Am J Kidney Dis. 2005;45(6):978–93.

28. Krapf R, Alpern RJ, Seldin DW. Clinical syndromes of metabolic acidosis. In: Seldin DW, Giebisch G, editors. The kidney. Philadelphia: Lippincott Williams & Wilkins; 2000. p. 2055–72.
29. Bidani A, DuBose TD. Acid–base regulation: cellular and whole body. In: Arieff AI, DeFronzo RA, editors. Fluid, electrolyte, and acid base disorders. New York: Churchill; 1995. p. 69.

Chapter 4
Etiologic Causes of Metabolic Acidosis II: Normal Anion Gap Acidoses

Thomas D. DuBose Jr.

Non-Anion Gap (Hyperchloremic) Metabolic Acidoses

Metabolic acidosis with a normal AG (hyperchloremic or non-AG acidosis) indicates that HCO_3^- in the plasma has been effectively replaced by Cl^-, and therefore, the AG does not change. The majority of disorders in this category can be attributed to either: (1) loss of bicarbonate from the gastrointestinal tract (diarrhea) or from the kidney (proximal RTA), or (2) inappropriately low kidney acid excretion (classical distal RTA [cDRTA], generalized distal RTA [type 4 RTA], or acute and chronic kidney disease). Hypokalemia may accompany gastrointestinal loss of HCO_3^-, proximal RTA, and cDRTA. Therefore, the major challenge in distinguishing these causes is to be able to define whether the response of kidney tubular function to the prevailing acidosis is appropriate acid excretion in the urine (consistent with gastrointestinal origin) or inappropriately low urine acid excretion (consistent with a kidney origin). The differential diagnosis of the non-gap acidoses is summarized in Table 4.1.

Diarrhea results in the loss of large quantities of HCO_3^- decomposed by reaction with organic acids. Because diarrheal stools contain a higher concentration of HCO_3^- and decomposed HCO_3^- than plasma, volume depletion and metabolic acidosis develop. Hypokalemia occurs because large quantities of K^+ are lost from stool and because volume depletion causes secondary hyperaldosteronism, which enhances K^+ secretion by the kidney collecting duct. Instead of an acid urine pH as might be anticipated with chronic diarrhea, a pH of 6.0 or more might be found. This occurs because chronic metabolic acidosis and hypokalemia each increases kidney ammonia (NH_3) buffer production that combines with protons (H^+) to form

T.D. DuBose Jr., M.D., M.A.C.P., F.A.S.N. (✉)
Section on General Internal Medicine, Wake Forest School of Medicine,
Medical Center Boulevard, Winston Salem, NC 27157, USA
e-mail: tdubose@wakehealth.edu

© Springer Science+Business Media New York 2016   27
D.E. Wesson (ed.), *Metabolic Acidosis*, DOI 10.1007/978-1-4939-3463-8_4

Table 4.1 Differential diagnosis of non-gap acidosis

Extra kidney causes
Diarrhea or other GI losses of bicarbonate (e.g., tube drainage)
Posttreatment of ketoacidosis (dilutional) (occasional: initial DKA)
Kidney causes not due to renal tubular acidosis
Ureteral diversion (e.g., ileal loop, ureterosigmoidostomy)
Progressive chronic kidney disease
Toluene ingestion (excretion of hippurate)
Drugs
With associated hypokalemia
Carbonic anhydrase inhibitors (acetazolamide and topiramate)
Amphotericin B
With associated hyperkalemia
Amiloride,
Triamterene,
Spironolactone,
Trimethoprim
With normal potassium
$CaCl_2$, $MgSO_4$
Cholestyramine
Exogenous acid loads (NH_4Cl, acidic amino acids—total parenteral nutrition, sulfur)
Post-hypocapnic state
Renal tubular acidosis
Low $[K^+]_p$
Type 1 (classical distal) RTA
Type 2 (proximal) RTA
Type 3 (mixed proximal and distal) RTA (carbonic anhydrase II deficiency)
High $[K^+]_p$
Type 4 (generalized distal RTA)
Hypoaldosteronism (hyporeninemic and isolated)
Aldosterone resistance
Voltage defect in collecting duct

ammonium (NH_4^+) for urine excretion. The resulting increase in urine NH_3/NH_4^+ buffer can increase urine pH. In the setting described, a urine pH of 6.0 or higher might erroneously suggest a non-kidney cause. Because urinary NH_4^+ excretion is typically low in patients with RTA and high in patients with diarrhea [1, 2], the level of urinary NH_4^+ excretion (not usually measured by clinical laboratories) in metabolic acidosis can be assessed indirectly [3] by calculating the urine anion gap (UAG), using the following equation [2]:

$$UAG = [Na^+ + K^+]_U - [Cl^-]_U \qquad (4.1)$$

where U denotes the urine concentration of these electrolytes. The rationale for using the UAG as a surrogate for ammonium excretion is that in chronic metabolic acidosis ammonium excretion should be elevated if kidney tubular function is intact. Therefore, the UAG should become progressively negative as the rate of ammonium excretion increases in response to acidosis or to acid loading [3, 4]. A negative UAG (more than −20 mEq/L) implies that sufficient NH_4^+ is present in the urine, as might occur with an extra kidney origin of the hyperchloremic acidosis. Conversely, urine estimated to contain little or no NH_4^+ has more $Na^+ + K^+$ than Cl^- (UAG is positive) [2–4], which indicates a kidney mechanism for the hyperchloremic acidosis, such as in cDRTA (with hypokalemia) or hypoaldosteronism with hyperkalemia. If a patient has ketonuria, drug anions (penicillins or aspirin), or toluene metabolites in the urine, this test is not reliable and should not be used.

In such circumstances the urinary ammonium concentration ($U_{NH_4^+}$) may be estimated more reliably from the urine osmolal gap, which is the difference in measured urine osmolality (U_{osm}), and the urine osmolality calculated from the urine $[Na^+ + K^+]$ and the urine urea and glucose (all expressed in mmol/L) [3]:

$$U_{NH_4^+} = 0.5(U_{Osm} - [2(Na^+ + K^+) + Urea + Glucose]_U \qquad (4.2)$$

Calculated urinary ammonium concentrations of 75 mEq/L or more would be anticipated if kidney tubular function is intact and the kidney is responding to the prevailing metabolic acidosis by increasing ammonium production and excretion. Values below 25 mEq/L denote inappropriately low urinary ammonium concentrations, suggesting the diagnosis of RTA.

Severe non-AG or hyperchloremic metabolic acidosis with hypokalemia may also occur in patients with ureteral diversion procedures. Because the ileum and the colon are both endowed with Cl^-/HCO_3^- exchangers, when the Cl^- from the urine enters the gut or pouch, the HCO_3^- concentration increases as a result of the exchange process and HCO_3^- is excreted [4]. Moreover, K^+ secretion is stimulated, which, together with HCO_3^- loss, can result in a non-AG (hyperchloremic) hypokalemic metabolic acidosis.

Loss of functioning kidney parenchyma in progressive kidney disease is associated with metabolic acidosis. Typically, the acidosis is a non-AG type when the GFR is between 20 and 50 mL/min but may convert to the typical high AG acidosis of uremia with more advanced chronic kidney disease, that is, when the GFR is less than 15–20 mL/min [5]. The principal defect in acidification of stage 3–4 CKD is that ammoniagenesis is reduced in proportion to the loss of functional kidney mass. Medullary NH_4^+ accumulation and trapping in the outer medullary collecting tubule may also be impaired [5]. Because of adaptive increases in K^+ secretion by the collecting duct and colon, the acidosis of chronic kidney disease is typically normokalemic [5]. Non-AG metabolic acidosis accompanied by hyperkalemia is almost always associated with a generalized dysfunction of the distal nephron [1, 2]. However, K^+-sparing diuretics (amiloride, triamterene), as well as pentamidine, cyclosporine, tacrolimus, nonsteroidal antiinflammatory drugs (NSAIDs), angiotensin converting enzyme (ACE) inhibitors, angiotensin II receptor blockers (ARBs), β-blockers, and heparin may cause hyperkalemia and a non-gap metabolic acidosis [1, 2]. Because hyperkalemia augments the development of acidosis by suppressing urinary net acid excretion, discontinuing these agents while reducing the serum K^+ allows ammonium production and excretion to increase, which will help repair the acidosis.

Disorders of Impaired Kidney Bicarbonate Reclamation: Proximal Renal Tubular Acidosis

Pathophysiology

The first phase of acidification by the nephron involves reabsorption of the filtered HCO_3^- so that 80 % of the filtered HCO_3^- is normally returned to the blood by the proximal convoluted tubule [1–3]. If the capacity of the proximal tubule is reduced, less of the filtered HCO_3^- is reabsorbed in this segment and more is delivered to the more distal segments (see Fig. 4.1). This increase in HCO_3^- delivery overwhelms the limited capacity for bicarbonate reabsorption by the distal nephron, and bicarbonaturia ensues, net acid excretion ceases, and metabolic acidosis follows. Enhanced Cl^- reabsorption, stimulated by ECF volume contraction, leading to replacement of lost $NaHCO_3$ with NaCl causes hyperchloremic (non-AG) chronic metabolic acidosis. With progressive metabolic acidosis and decreased serum HCO_3^- levels, the filtered HCO_3^- load declines progressively. As plasma HCO_3^- concentration decreases, the defective HCO_3^- reabsorption more completely absorbs the lower filtered load of HCO_3^- so that the absolute amount of HCO_3^- entering the distal nephron eventually reaches the level approximating the distal HCO_3^- delivery in normal individuals (at the normal threshold). At this point the reduced quantity of HCO_3^- entering the distal nephron can be reabsorbed completely, so urine pH declines. As a consequence, the serum HCO_3^- concentration usually reaches a nadir of 15–18 mEq/L, and the systemic acidosis no longer progresses. Therefore, in proximal RTA, in the steady state, the serum HCO_3^- is usually about 15–18 mEq/L and the urine pH acid (<5.5). With bicarbonate administration, the amount of bicarbonate in the urine increases the fractional excretion of bicarbonate ($FE_{HCO_3^-}$) to 15 % or more, and the urine pH becomes alkaline [1], and the diagnosis of proximal RTA can be made.

Proximal RTA can present in one of three ways (summarized in Fig. 4.1): one in which acidification is the only defective function, one in which there is a more generalized proximal tubule dysfunction with multi-transporter abnormalities (most common), and as a part of a mixed variety of RTA (type 3). Inheritance patterns for isolated proximal RTA include autosomal recessive and autosomal dominant. Isolated pure bicarbonate wasting is typical of autosomal recessive proximal RTA with accompanying ocular abnormalities and has been defined as a number of mis-

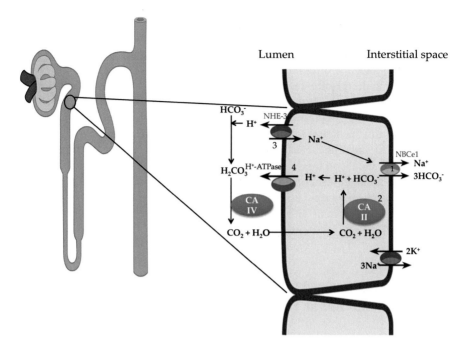

Fig. 4.1 Model of acidification in the proximal convoluted tubule. Numbers refer to unique defects in specific transporters responsible for defective bicarbonate absorption and bicarbonaturia typical of proximal RTA: 1. Autosomal recessive mutation of NBCe1/*SLC4A4* located on B-L membrane. 2. Carbonic anhydrase II deficiency causing osteopetrosis, mixed proximal/distal RTA (Type III RTA). 3. Autosomal dominant mutation of NHE-3. 4. Inherited defect of the H^+-ATPase (has not been described in association with proximal RTA)

sense mutations of the gene *SLCA4* that encodes for the basolateral transporter, NBCe1. A rare variant, inherited as an autosomal dominant trait, has been described and appears to be a mutation of the gene that encodes the apical Na^+/H^+ exchanger, NHE-3, and has been reported to be associated with short stature. Familial disorders associated with proximal RTA include: cystinosis, tyrosinemia, hereditary fructose intolerance, galactosemia, glycogen storage disease type 1, Wilson's disease, and Lowe's syndrome.

Additionally, features of both proximal RTA (bicarbonate wasting), and distal acidification abnormalities are evident in patients with autosomal recessive RTA (mixed proximal and distal, or type 3 RTA) that has been attributed to a defect in the *CA2* gene that encodes for carbonic anhydrase II (CAII), an intracellular form of the enzyme distributed to the proximal tubule and other distal tubule segments [1]. The phenotype includes osteopetrosis, and ocular abnormalities.

The majority of cases of proximal RTA fit into the category of generalized proximal tubule dysfunction with multi-transport abnormalities manifest as glycosuria, aminoaciduria, hypercitraturia, and phosphaturia, and referred to as *Fanconi's syndrome*.

Although proximal RTA is more common in children, the most common causes of acquired proximal RTA in adults are multiple myeloma, in which increased excretion of immunoglobulin light chains injures the proximal tubule epithelium, and chemotherapeutic drug injury of the proximal tubule (e.g., ifosfamide). RTA due to ifosfamide toxicity, lead intoxication, and cystinosis is more common in children. Carbonic anhydrase inhibitors cause pure bicarbonate wasting but not Fanconi's syndrome. Topiramate, widely used in the prevention of migraine headaches, or for treatment of a seizure disorder is a potent carbonic anhydrase inhibitor, and is an important cause of non-AG metabolic acidosis. Approximately 15–25 % of patients on topiramate will manifest a stable non-gap metabolic acidosis due to a mixed form of RTA with features of both proximal and distal RTA (type 3). This phenotype occurs because the enzyme carbonic anhydrase II is present in both the proximal and distal tubules, and subsides when topiramate is discontinued.

Disorders of Impaired Net Acid Excretion with Hypokalemia: Classical Distal Renal Tubule Acidosis

Pathophysiology

The mechanisms involved in the pathogenesis of hypokalemic cDRTA (type 1 RTA) have been more clearly elucidated by appreciation of the genetic and molecular bases of the inherited forms of this disease in the last two decades. Most studies suggest that the inherited forms of cDRTA are due to inherited defects in either the basolateral HCO_3^-/Cl^- exchanger (encoded by the gene *SLC4A1*), or subunits of the H^+-ATPase (encoded by the *ATP6V1B1 or ATP6V0A4 genes, respectively*) localized to the Type A intercalated cell of the collecting duct (Fig. 4.2).

While the classical finding is an inability to acidify the urine maximally (to a pH of <5.5) in the face of systemic acidosis, attention to urine ammonium excretion rather than urine pH alone is necessary to diagnose this disorder [1, 2]. The pathogenesis of the acidification defect in most patients is evident by the response of the urine PCO_2 to sodium bicarbonate infusion. When normal subjects are given large infusions of sodium bicarbonate to produce a high HCO_3^- excretion, distal nephron H^+ secretion leads to the generation of a high PCO_2 in the kidney medulla and final urine [8, 9]. The magnitude of the urinary PCO_2 (often referred to as the *urine minus blood* PCO_2 or $U-B$ PCO_2) can be used as an index of distal nephron H^+ secretory capacity [6–9]. The $U-B$ PCO_2 is generally subnormal in classical hypokalemic distal RTA, with the notable exception of amphotericin B-induced distal RTA, which remains the most common example of the "gradient" defect [7, 9, 10].

Patients with impaired collecting duct H^+ secretion and cDRTA exhibit uniformly low excretory rates of NH_4^+ when the degree of systemic acidosis is taken into

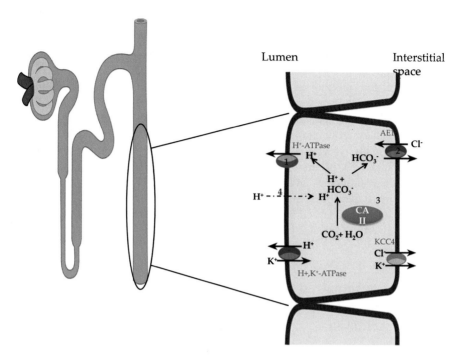

Fig. 4.2 Type A intercalated cell of cortical collecting duct and reported causes of distal renal tubular acidosis. 1. Inherited or acquired defect of the H⁺-ATPase. Autosomal recessive mutations of *ATP6V1B1* with deafness and of *ATP6V04* without deafness have been reported. Defects in the H⁺-ATPase may be acquired in Sjögren's syndrome. 2. Autosomal dominant mutations of *SLC4A1* cause an abnormality of the basolateral HCO_3^-/Cl^- exchanger. 3. Carbonic anhydrase II deficiency is associated with mixed (Type III) proximal and distal RTA. 4. Inherited or acquired disorders resulting in backleak of H⁺ have been reported. The acquired defect best described is that caused by the antibiotic amphotericin B

account [1, 2, 11]. Low NH_4^+ excretion equates with inappropriately low regeneration of HCO_3^- by the kidney, which indicates that the kidney is responsible for causing or perpetuating the chronic metabolic acidosis. Low NH_4^+ excretion in classical hypokalemic distal RTA occurs because of the failure to trap NH_4^+ in the medullary collecting duct as a result of higher than normal tubule fluid pH in this segment and loss of the disequilibrium pH (pH>6.0) [12].

Medullary interstitial disease, which commonly occurs in conjunction with distal RTA, may impair NH_4^+ excretion by interrupting the medullary countercurrent system for NH_4^+ [1, 2, 13, 14]. The complete form of classical distal RTA is manifest by a non-AG acidosis without treatment. The clinical spectrum of complete cDRTA may include stunted growth, hypercalciuria, hypocitraturia, osteopenia, nephrolithiasis, and nephrocalcinosis, all a direct consequence of the chronic non-AG metabolic acidosis. The dissolution of bone is due to calcium resorption and mobilization from bone in response to the acidosis [1] and through activation of the pH sensitive

G-protein coupled receptor, OGR1, which resides in bone [15]. Other common electrolyte abnormalities, not due to acidosis include hypokalemia, hypernatremia and salt wasting, and polyuria due to nephrogenic diabetes insipidus. The hypokalemia may be due to a signaling pathway involving activation and release of PGE2 by β-intercalated cells that directly communicate to enhance sodium absorption and potassium secretion by activation of the epithelial sodium channel (ENaC) and BK channels in collecting duct principal cells. Because chronic metabolic acidosis also decreases kidney production of citrate [1, 2, 11], the resulting hypocitraturia in combination with hypercalciuria increases urinary stone formation and nephrocalcinosis. Distal RTA occurs frequently in patients with Sjögren's syndrome and because of autoantibodies and infiltration of lymphocytes, is due to the inability to traffic and insert the H^+-ATPase into the apical membrane properly [16]. The numerous causes of both inherited and acquired defects resulting in classical distal RTA are summarized in Table 4.2.

Disorders of Impaired Net Acid Excretion with Hyperkalemia: Generalized Distal Nephron Dysfunction (Type 4 Renal Tubular Acidosis)

The coexistence of hyperkalemia and a non-gap metabolic acidosis indicates a generalized dysfunction in the cortical and medullary collecting tubules [1, 2]. Hyperkalemia is an important mediator of the kidney response to acid–base balance, because it independently reduces ammonium production and excretion. Chronic hyperkalemia decreases ammonium production in the proximal tubule and whole kidney, inhibits absorption of NH_4^+ in the mTAL, reduces medullary interstitial concentrations of NH_4^+ and NH_3, and decreases entry of NH_4^+ and NH_3 into the medullary collecting duct, all leading to a marked reduction in urinary ammonium excretion [1, 2]. The potential for development of a hyperchloremic metabolic acidosis is greatly augmented when a reduction in functional kidney mass (GFR of <60 mL/min) coexists with hyperkalemia or when aldosterone deficiency or resistance is present.

Drug-Induced Kidney Tub ular Secretory Defects

Impaired Renin–Aldosterone Elaboration

Drugs may impair renin or aldosterone elaboration or cause mineralocorticoid resistance in patients with CKD, and produce effects that mimic the clinical manifestations of the acidification defect seen in the generalized form of distal RTA with hyperkalemia. Examples include NSAIDs or COX-2 inhibitors [17], spironolactone and eplerenone, β-adrenergic antagonists, heparin, and ACE inhibitors and ARBs.

Table 4.2 Disorders associated with classical hypokalemic distal RTA primary

Familial	
1. Autosomal dominant	
a. Abnormality of the basolateral HCO_3^-/Cl^- exchanger (AE-1) due to *SLC4A1* mutation	
2. Autosomal recessive	
a. Deficiency or abnormality of the H^+-ATPase Autosomal recessive *ATP6V1B1* mutation with deafness Autosomal recessive *ATP6V0A4* mutation with or without deafness b. Carbonic anhydrase II deficiency—mixed PRTA–DRTA	
Endemic	
Northeastern Thailand	
Acquired defect of the H^+-ATPase	
Sjögren's syndrome	
Secondary to systemic disorders	
Autoimmune diseases	
Hyperglobulinemic purpura	Fibrosing alveolitis
Cryoglobulinemia	Chronic active hepatitis
Sjögren's syndrome	Primary biliary cirrhosis
Thyroiditis	Polyarthritis nodosa
HIV nephropathy	
Hypercalciuria and nephrocalcinosis	
Primary hyperparathyroidism	Vitamin D intoxication
Hyperthyroidism	Idiopathic hypercalciuria
Medullary sponge kidney	Wilson disease
Fabry disease	Hereditary fructose intolerance
X-linked hypophosphatemia	Hereditary sensorineural deafness
Drug and toxin induced disease	
Amphotericin B	Cyclamate
Mercury	
Vanadate	Lithium
Hepatic cirrhosis	Classic analgesic nephropathy
Ifosfamide	Foscarnet
Topiramate	Acetazolamide
Tubulointerstitial diseases	
Balkan nephropathy	Kidney transplantation
Chronic pyelonephritis	Leprosy
Obstructive uropathy	Jejunoileal bypass with hyperoxaluria
Vesicoureteral reflux	
Associated with genetically transmitted diseases	
Ehlers–Danlos syndrome	Hereditary elliptocytosis
Sickle cell anemia	Marfan syndrome
Medullary cystic disease	Jejunal bypass with hyperoxaluria
Hereditary sensorineural deafness	Carnitine palmitoyltransferase I
Osteopetrosis with carbonic anhydrase II deficiency	

Voltage Defect of Collecting Duct

Autosomal recessive PHA-1. This disorder is the result of a loss-of-function mutation of the gene that encodes one of the α-, β-, or γ-subunits of the ENaC [18–22].
Typically, children with PHA-1 also manifest vomiting, hyponatremia, failure to
thrive, and respiratory distress [21, 23], and respond to a high salt intake and correction of the hyperkalemia.

Amiloride and triamterene may be associated with hyperkalemia, because these
potassium-sparing diuretics occupy and thus block the apical Na⁺-selective channel
(ENaC) in the collecting duct principal cell. Occupation of ENaC inhibits Na⁺
absorption and reduces the negative transepithelial voltage, which alters the driving
force for K⁺ secretion (Fig. 4.3 displays the pathophysiology of a prototypical voltage defect in the CCT).

The calcineurin inhibitors cyclosporine A and tacrolimus may be associated with
hyperkalemia in the transplant recipient as a result of inhibition of the basolateral
Na⁺-K⁺-ATPase and the consequent decrease in intracellular [K⁺] and the transepithelial potential, which together reduce the driving force for K⁺ secretion (see Fig.
4.3) [17]. Calcineurin inhibitors may also inhibit K⁺ secretion by directly interfering

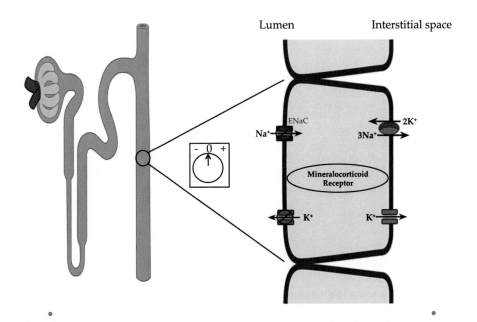

Fig. 4.3 Definition of voltage defect in the cortical collecting duct principal cell. Loss of function
of the Na⁺ channel, ENaC, prevents the generation of a lumen-negative transepithelial potential,
therefore, negating the favorable voltage for K⁺ secretion into the lumen (similarly, H⁺ secretion by
the neighboring Type A intercalated cell is also impaired). Calcineurin inhibitors may cause a voltage defect by inhibition of the B-L Na⁺,K⁺-ATPase or by inhibition of the ROMK channel on the
apical membrane. Most voltage defects cause hyperkalemic non-gap metabolic acidosis, therefore

with the K channel, ROMK [24]. An additional explanation for the association of hyperkalemia, volume expansion and hypertension, a syndrome that resembles the phenotype of familial hyperkalemic hypertension or PHA-2, is enhanced activity of NCC in the DCT [25].

Disorders of Impaired Net Acid Excretion and Impaired Bicarbonate Reclamation with Normokalemia: Acidosis of Progressive Kidney Failure

The metabolic acidosis of CKD associated with chronically reduced GFR is initially hyperchloremic (GFR in the range of 20–30 mL/min) but may convert to the high AG variety as kidney insufficiency progresses and GFR falls below 15 mL/min [2, 5]. Unlike patients with classical distal RTA, patients with primary kidney disease have a normal ability to lower the urine pH during acidosis [5]. The net distal H^+ secretory capacity is qualitatively normal and can be increased by buffer availability in the form of PO_4^{3-} or by nonreabsorbable anions. Thus, the principal defect is an inability to produce or to excrete NH_4^+ sufficient to match net endogenous acid production. Consequently, the kidneys cannot quantitatively excrete all the metabolic acids produced daily, and net positive acid balance supervenes [5].

Evidence continues to indicate that chronic acidosis in patients with CKD is deleterious and accelerates CKD progression [26, 27] and augments dissolution of bone [2], and impaired hydroxylation of 25-hydroxycholecalciferol [2, 5], causing kidney osteodystrophy. Furthermore, the chronic acidosis also causes sarcopenia from enhanced skeletal muscle protein degradation with subsequent loss of muscle strength.

References

1. Laski ME, Wesson DE. Lactic acidosis. In: DuBose TD, Hamm LL, editors. Acid–base and electrolyte disorders: a companion to Brenner and Rector's the kidney. Philadelphia: Saunders; 2002. p. 68–83.
2. DuBose TD, McDonald GA. Renal tubular acidosis. In: DuBose TD, Hamm LL, editors. Acid–base and electrolyte disorders: a companion to Brenner and Rector's the kidney. Philadelphia: Saunders; 2002. p. 189–206.
3. Goraya N, Simoni J, Jo CH, Wesson DE. A comparison of treating metabolic acidosis in CKD stage 4 hypertensive kidney disease with fruits and vegetables or sodium bicarbonate. Clin J Am Soc Nephrol. 2013;8:371–81.
4. Krapf R, Alpern RJ, Seldin DW. Clinical syndromes of metabolic acidosis. In: Seldin DW, Giebisch G, editors. The kidney. Philadelphia: Lippincott Williams & Wilkins; 2000. p. 2055–72.
5. John M, Mallal S. Hyperlactatemia syndromes in people with HIV infection. Curr Opin Infect Dis. 2002;15:23–9.

6. Cote HC, Brumme ZL, Craib KJ, et al. Changes in mitochondrial DNA as a marker of nucleo-side toxicity in HIV-infected patients. N Engl J Med. 2002;346:811–20.
7. Lalau JD, Race JM. Lactic acidosis in metformin therapy. Drugs. 1999;58 Suppl 1:55–60.
8. Calabrese AT, Coley KC, DaPos SV, et al. Evaluation of prescribing practices: risk of lactic acidosis with metformin therapy. Arch Intern Med. 2002;162:434–7.
9. Romanski SA, McMahon MM. Metabolic acidosis and thiamine deficiency. Mayo Clin Proc. 1999;74:259–63.
10. Luft FC. Lactic acidosis update for critical care clinicians. J Am Soc Nephrol. 2001;12 Suppl 17:S15–9.
11. Gerard Y, Maulin L, Yazdanpanah Y, et al. Symptomatic hyperlactatemia: an emerging complication of antiretroviral therapy. AIDS. 2000;14:2723–30.
12. Uchida H, Yamamoto H, Kisaki Y, et al. D-Lactic acidosis in short-bowel syndrome managed with antibiotics and probiotics. J Pediatr Surg. 2004;39:634–6.
13. Jorens PG, Demey HE, Schepens PJ, et al. Unusual D-lactic acid acidosis from propylene glycol metabolism in overdose. J Toxicol Clin Toxicol. 2004;42:163–9.
14. Lalive PH, Hadengue A, Mensi N, Burkhard PR. Recurrent encephalopathy after small bowel resection. Implication of D-lactate. Rev Neurol (Paris). 2001;157:679–81.
15. Whitney GM, Szerlip HM. Acid–base disorders in the critical care setting. In: DuBose TD, Hamm LL, editors. Acid–base and electrolyte disorders: a companion to Brenner and Rector's the kidney. Philadelphia: Saunders; 2002. p. 165–87.
16. Halperin ML, Kamel KS, Cherney DZ. Ketoacidosis. In: DuBose TD, Hamm LL, editors. Acid–base and electrolyte disorders: a companion to Brenner and Rector's the kidney. Philadelphia: Saunders; 2002. p. 67–82.
17. Umpierrez GE, DiGirolamo M, Tuvlin JA, et al. Differences in metabolic and hormonal milieu in diabetic- and alcohol-induced ketoacidosis. J Crit Care. 2000;15:52–9.
18. DuBose TD, Alpern RJ. Renal tubular acidosis. In: The metabolic and molecular bases of inherited disease. New York: McGraw-Hill; 2001. p. 4983–5021.
19. Proudfoot AT, Krenzelok EP, Brent J, Vale JA. Does urine alkalinization increase salicylate elimination? If so, why? Toxicol Rev. 2003;22:129–36.
20. Brent J. Fomepizole for ethylene glycol and methanol poisoning. N Engl J Med. 2009;360:2216–23.
21. Fraser AD. Clinical toxicologic implications of ethylene glycol and glycolic acid poisoning. Ther Drug Monit. 2002;24:232–8.
22. Velez LI, Shepherd G, Lee YC, Keyes DC. Ethylene glycol ingestion treated only with fomepizole. J Med Toxicol. 2007;3:125–8.
23. Mizock BA, Belyaev S, Mecher C. Unexplained metabolic acidosis in critically ill patients: the role of pyroglutamic acid. Intensive Care Med. 2004;30:502–5.
24. Wilson KC, Reardon C, Farber HW. Propylene glycol toxicity in a patient receiving intravenous diazepam. N Engl J Med. 2000;343:815.
25. Zar T, Yusufzai I, Sullivan A, Graeber C. Acute kidney injury, hyperosmolality and metabolic acidosis associated with lorazepam. Nat Clin Pract Nephrol. 2007;3:515–20.
26. Loniewski I, Wesson DE. Bicarbonate therapy for prevention of chronic kidney disease progression. Kidney Int. 2014;85:529–35.
27. Goraya N, Simoni J, Jo C-H, Wesson DE. Treatment of metabolic acidosis in individuals with stage 3 CKD with fruits and vegetables or oral $NaHCO_3$ reduces urine angiotensinogen and preserves GFR. Kidney Int. 2014;86:1031–8.

Chapter 5
The Use of Bedside Urinary Parameters in the Evaluation of Metabolic Acidosis

Daniel Batlle, Khurram Saleem, and Nitin Relia

Introduction

The pathophysiologic approach to the evaluation of metabolic acidosis and the importance of a complete evaluation of urine acid excretion and its main components (ammonium and titratable acids) has been discussed in a previous chapter. In this article we discuss the evaluation of the kidney response to metabolic acidosis at the bedside using basic tools as urine pH, urine anion gap, and urine bicarbonate and discuss their interpretation and limitations. The use of provocative tests to evaluate distal acidification in patients suspected of distal renal tubular acidosis (DRTA) is also discussed.

Urine pH

Urine pH depends mainly on the concentration of HCO_3^-: the higher the urine concentration of HCO_3^-, the higher the urine pH. In normal subjects urine pH is approximately 6.0 for the majority of measurements during a 24-h period [1]. This reflects that the urine normally contains little HCO_3^- and therefore $UHCO_3^-$ can be considered negligible at this urine pH. Depending on the acid–base status, the range of urine pH varies widely from 4.5 to 8.0 [2]. Urine pH should be measured in a

D. Batlle, M.D. • N. Relia, M.D.
Division of Nephrology and Hypertension, Northwestern University Feinberg School of Medicine, 320 E. Superior, Chicago, IL 60611, USA
e-mail: d-batlle@northwestern.edu; docnrelia@gmail.com

K. Saleem, M.D. (✉)
Department of Nephrology, Northwestern Memorial Hospital,
710 North Fairbanks Court Suite 4-500, Chicago, IL 60611, USA
e-mail: Khurram.saleem@northwestern.edu

© Springer Science+Business Media New York 2016
D.E. Wesson (ed.), *Metabolic Acidosis*, DOI 10.1007/978-1-4939-3463-8_5

freshly voided sample, preferably in the morning, and collection under mineral oil has been traditionally recommended to prevent CO_2 diffusion. This time honored practice for research purposes has been difficult to follow in the busy hospital setting. The need for collecting urine under mineral oil has been recently challenged [3]. In a recent study of 97 random acidic urinary samples (pH < 7.0), urine pH was not substantially altered when studied under mineral oil as compared with 5 min of vigorous shaking [3].

The correlation between urine ΔpH after CO_2 loss from shaking and the corresponding baseline pH in oil-free acidic urine samples ($n = 97$ samples) is shown in Fig. 5.1. The graph of the relationship between these variables is a reversed parabolic curve, pointing to a tendency for smaller increases in urine pH (after CO_2 loss) in samples with lower than higher urine at baseline pH. This finding suggests that, unlike the situation for alkaline urine (pH > 7.0), collection of urine under oil is not necessary for acidic urine [3]. While this is good information, the problem still remains that one does not know if the urine is going to be acidic or alkaline until the pH is measured. Moreover, the effect of prolonged exposure to air on urine pH was not studied in this report [3]. Collecting urine with mineral oil, in our opinion, should continue to be recommended for measuring urine pH and PCO_2. When not possible it seems reasonable to measure urine pH as soon as possible (within 1 h or so) after freshly voiding urine is collected.

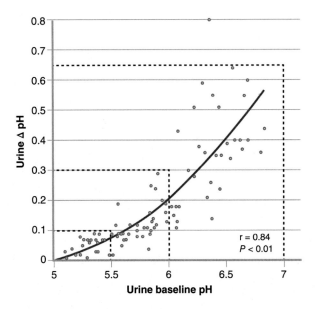

Fig. 5.1 Correlation between the urine pH after CO_2 loss because of shaking and the corresponding baseline pH oil-free acidic urine samples ($n = 97$). *Dotted lines* at pH values of 5.5, 6.0, and 7.0 reveal the degree of urine pH by 0.1, 0.3, and 0.65, respectively. Modified from Yi et al. CJASN 2012;7(8):1222–16

Limitations and Caveats in the Interpretation of Urine pH

The concept that urine pH>5.5 in the setting of metabolic acidosis is an indication of defective H^+ secretion by the distal nephron originated from observations that patients with the classic form of distal RTA could not lower urine pH below this level even under conditions of severe metabolic acidosis [4–6]. The urine pH alone, however is not sufficient to evaluate the intactness of collecting tubule H^+ secretion. This requires information on acid excretion, namely NH_4^+ (see below). Moreover, other caveats, must be taken into account for the use of urine pH as an index for distal H^+ secretion.

One caveat is that distal Na^+ delivery must be adequate [6, 7]. Low Na^+ delivery to the distal nephron impairs maximal distal acidification in response to acidemia [6]. When Na^+ excretion is increased by salt replacement, urine pH falls maximally and acid excretion increases with improvement in the metabolic acidosis [6]. A clue to the diagnosis of chronic laxative abuse as the cause of metabolic acidosis is the finding of low urine Na^+, which may be less than 10 mEq/day. Patients with hepatorenal syndrome likewise may not be able to acidify the urine maximally owing to lack of adequate distal Na^+ delivery.

The concentration of urine buffers such as NH_4^+ affects urine pH [8, 9]. Under conditions of maximal stimulation of H^+ excretion urine pH may not be lower than 5.5. If there is a marked increase in NH_3^+ formation, secreted H^+ is buffered to form NH_4^+ and its concentration in the urine is actually low, this being reflected by a relatively high urine pH [2, 8, 9]. In this setting, a urine pH above 5.5 does not imply that a defect in distal H^+ secretion is present and the associated high NH_4^+ excretion rules out such defect.

The urine pH should be therefore interpreted in the context of the level of NH_4^+ excretion (see Table 5.1). The finding of a urine pH>5.5 in the presence of metabolic acidosis is consistent with the diagnosis of RTA but NH_4^+ excretion needs to be reduced for this diagnosis (Table 5.1). Patients with hyperkalemia and aldosterone deficiency (type 4 RTA) have decreased NH_4^+ excretion as a result of lack of aldosterone and

Table 5.1 Urine pH, NH_4^+, and UAG in various causes of metabolic acidosis

	Urine pH	Urine NH_4^+	Urine anion gap
DRTA (classic)	>5.5	Decreased	Increased (positive)
Metabolic acidosis (i.e., mild diarrhea)	<5.5	Increased	Decreased (negative)
Metabolic acidosis (severe protracted diarrhea)	>5.5	Much increased	Much decreased (very negative)
Type 4 RTA	<5.5	Much decreased	Much increased (very positive)
Hyperkalemic distal RTA	>5.5	Much decreased	Much increased (very positive)
Advanced CKD	<5.5	Much decreased	Much increased (very positive)

hyperkalemia which both suppress ammonium formation [10]. Such patients have low urine pH (Table 5.1) [10, 11] because urine NH_4^+ is so low in the collecting tubule that even a low rate of H^+ secretion translates into a low urine pH.

Patients with hyperkalemic DRTA, not caused by aldosterone deficiency, cannot lower urine pH and ammonium excretion is decreased (Table 5.1) [12].

Urine Bicarbonate

Urine bicarbonate excretion is usually very low and urine organic anions such as citrate represent the main mode of base excretion. During metabolic acidosis and with chronic acid loads there is a decrease in base excretion in the form of citrate and other organic anions [13]. Low urine citrate might better reflect adaptation to metabolic acidosis than low urine bicarbonate. This is because low urine citrate suggests kidney retention of potential base whereas urine HCO_3 is already low under baseline conditions in most patients under normal conditions because of near complete reabsorption.

Provided that both urine pH and PCO_2 are available one can calculate the urine HCO_3^- concentration using a derivation of the Henderson–Hasselbalch equation as shown below:

$$\text{Urine HCO}_3^- = \alpha\,PCO_2 \times 10^{pH-pK}$$

where α is the solubility coefficient for urine PCO_2 (0.03).

Urine Na^+ and K^+ should ideally be included to calculate urine pK and take into account the ionic strength of the urine, according to the formula:

$$pK = 6.33 - 0.5\sqrt{Na} + K$$

This, however, is not really necessary as shown by a recent study showing no significant difference in urinary HCO_3^- whether pK was calculated including urinary Na and K or simply using a pK of 6.1 (the pK of the HCO_3^- buffer). The latter formula is as follows:

$$\text{Urine HCO}_3^- = 0.03 \times PCO_2 \times 10^{pH-6.1}$$

Using this formula only urine PCO_2 and urine pH are needed to calculate urine HCO_3^-. Under conditions of eucapnia (normal blood PCO_2) urine PCO_2 is about 40 mmHg [14]. Therefore, when urine PCO_2 is not available (as it is often the case) one can assume that urine PCO_2 is 40 mmHg. This approach is practical because clinical laboratories do not routinely measure urine PCO_2. Ideally, however, urine PCO_2 should be measured as it maybe much lower or higher than blood PCO_2. A urine pH<6.5 denotes trivial amounts of HCO_3^- in the urine. An alkaline urine pH (>7.0) indicates bicarbonaturia.

Urine Electrolytes and the Urine Anion Gap

Urine Na^+, K^+, and Cl^- are needed to calculate the urine anion gap. In addition, urine Na^+ provides information of distal Na^+ delivery which is critical for optimal collecting tubule H^+ secretion as noted above. In the presence of metabolic acidosis, NH_4^+ is the most important component of urine acid excretion. Urine NH_4^+ is usually not measured in clinical laboratories but can be inferred by calculating the urine anion gap in patients with a hyperchloremic metabolic acidosis [15]. The principle is similar to that of the plasma anion gap, namely, that the sum of all anions must equal the sum of all cations. The unmeasured anions (UA) include sulfate, phosphate, and organic anions. Not routinely measured cations (UC) include NH_4^+, Ca^{++}, and Mg^{++}.

Including anions and cations other than those routinely measured (Cl^-, HCO_3^-, and Na^+ and K^+) it follows that:

$$(Cl^- + HCO_3^-) + UA = (Na^+ + K^+) + UC$$
$$\text{or } UA - UC = \left(Na^+ + K^+\right) - \left(Cl^- + HCO_3^-\right)$$

The urine anion gap is calculated by the formula:

$$\text{Urine anion gap} = (Na^+ + K^+) - (Cl^- + HCO_3^-)$$

If urine pH is <6.5, urine HCO_3^- does not need to be included as it can be considered negligible. Thus,

$$\text{Urine anion gap} = (Na^+ + K^+) - Cl^- = UA - UC$$

NH_4^+ is by far the predominant cation in the setting of metabolic acidosis and its excretion can be indirectly estimated through the urinary anion gap (Fig. 5.2) [15]. Because NH_4^+, the major unmeasured cation, increases markedly in the presence of metabolic acidosis, the UAG changes predictably and in this setting provides a rough estimate of urine NH_4^+.

The urine anion gap will be low (usually a negative value) if there is a decrease in unmeasured anions or an increase in unmeasured cations (e.g., NH_4^+). The latter occurs when NH_4 formation is increased to compensate for metabolic acidosis [15]. Conversely, the urine anion gap will be increased (usually a positive value) if there is a decrease in unmeasured cations (e.g., NH_4^+).

It should be noted that the utility of the UAG centers around the evaluation of metabolic acidosis. The urine anion gap can be decreased (typically a negative value) in diarrhea associated metabolic acidosis whereas it is typically increased (typically a positive value) in DRTA [15]. Patients with DRTA have a positive urine anion gap because NH_4^+ excretion is low as a result of failure to secrete H^+ in the distal nephron. By contrast, in diarrheal states associated with metabolic acidosis, the urine anion gap is negative, reflecting the fact that NH_4^+ excretion is

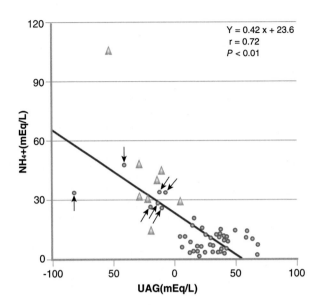

Fig. 5.2 Urinary ammonium (NH$_4$$^+$) in relation to the urinary anion gap (UAG). Thirty-eight patients with altered distal urinary acidification are represented by *open circles*; seven normal subjects receiving ammonium chloride, *closed circles*; and eight patients with hyperchloremic metabolic acidosis associated with diarrhea, *triangles*. Modified from Batlle DC, Hizon M, Cohen E, Gutterman C, Gupta R. The use of the urinary anion gap in the diagnosis of hyperchloremic metabolic acidosis. N Engl J Med 1988;318:594–9

appropriately increased [15, 16]. Information regarding NH$_4$$^+$ excretion from subjects with proximal RTA is limited. NH$_4$$^+$ excretion in proximal RTA is not reduced compared to control subjects [17, 18]. The response to a 3-day acid loading test with NH$_4$Cl was evaluated in eight patients with isolated proximal RTA and in 10 healthy control subjects [19]. In the basal state, all subjects with proximal RTA had NH$_4$$^+$ excretion rates similar to control subjects, suggesting normal kidney NH$_4$$^+$ handling. On the third day of acid loading, however, NH$_4$$^+$ excretion rates in proximal RTA patients were significantly lower than in controls, demonstrating an impairment in maximal urinary NH$_4$$^+$ excretion [19]. Given this finding and although the urine anion gap was not reported, it is likely that in proximal RTA the UAG is not as negative as in controls with metabolic acidosis, and actually could be slightly positive. In distal RTA, the urine anion gap is consistently positive without exceptions and very much increased (Figure. 5.2) [15].

The urine anion gap is also useful in helping the clinician to identify the presence of chronic respiratory alkalosis. Chronic respiratory alkalosis presents with hyperchloremia and hypobicarbonatemia [2, 20]. Consequently, the clinician might mistakenly diagnose chronic metabolic acidosis in a patient with chronic respiratory alkalosis, particularly when blood pH and blood PCO$_2$ are not available. The urine anion gap helps distinguish between chronic respiratory alkalosis and chronic metabolic acidosis. A positive urine anion gap in the presence of hyperchloremia and hypobicarbonatemia suggests either chronic respiratory alkalosis or DRTA [2].

Because DRTA is relatively rare and chronic respiratory alkalosis is frequently seen in hospitalized patients, the urine anion gap is a helpful way to distinguish metabolic acidosis from respiratory alkalosis. In chronic respiratory alkalosis, the urine anion gap is positive owing to suppressed NH_4^+ excretion as an adaptive response to chronic alkalemia [2]. By contrast, the urine anion gap is expected to be decreased (negative) with chronic metabolic acidosis when NH_4^+ formation and excretion are appropriately increased. The acidosis associated with chronic kidney failure (or advanced CKD) is largely due to a decrease in NH_4^+ excretion. Normally an acid load results in a several-fold increase in NH_4^+ excretion with a more modest increase in titratable acid excretion. By contrast, in advanced CKD, despite the prevailing systemic acidosis, there is a failure to increase NH_4^+ excretion to the levels found in normal subjects with metabolic acidosis [2]. Even when factored for GFR, NH_4^+ excretion in patients with advanced CKD fails to increase appropriately [21]. Accordingly, the urine anion gap is expected to be increased (positive) in patients with CKD even in the presence of metabolic acidosis (Table 5.1).

Although, the urinary anion gap roughly reflects urine NH_4^+ excretion, it is not a precise diagnostic index and does have limitations [15, 16]. For example, the urine anion gap may be decreased (i.e., negative) if the urine contained large amounts of unusual cations such as lithium. Conversely, the UAG may be increased (i.e., positive) if the urine contained certain anionic antibiotics such as carbenicillin.

These situations, however, are unusual and can be suspected based on clinical information. It is important to emphasize that the use of the UAG should be limited to the evaluation of NH_4^+ when plasma bicarbonate is reduced. One situation where the UAG can be misleading is the metabolic acidosis caused by ketoacidosis. In this situation, the UAG is likely to be increased (positive) despite a high excretion of NH_4^+ due to the presence of large amounts of ketone anions, which increases the UAG [13]. In this setting, the UAG would greatly underestimate NH_4^+ excretion. The UAG could also be affected by toluene intoxication because of the presence of hippurate [16, 22]. Despite these caveats, the urine anion gap is a useful bedside index of NH_4^+ excretion in patients with acidosis. Clearly it helps distinguish the common causes of metabolic acidosis due to diarrheal states from distal RTA. Moreover, it helps identify the presence of a chronic respiratory alkalosis as noted above.

Provocative Tests of Distal Acidification

Ammonium Chloride Test

If metabolic acidosis is not present, the acidifying agent ammonium chloride can be given orally in a dose of 0.1 g/kg body weight daily for 3–5 days [23]. A single dose of the same cumulative amount can also be given and urine is then collected hourly from 2 to 8 h. In healthy subjects, urine pH falls below 5.5 (usually <5.0) usually by the first day after NH_4Cl administration. By day three, NH_4^+ excretion increases at least three- to fivefold. Some others have suggested that 1-day NH$_4$Cl challenge only to make the test more practical. This approach, however, is not as reliable as the 3-day test. We think the 3-day test gives more reliable results and is preferable in that it allows time for a maximal increase in NH$_4^+$ excretion. An alternative acidifying agent is calcium chloride (2 mEq/kg of body weight orally), which gives results similar to ammonium chloride. It can be used in patients who cannot tolerate ammonium chloride due to nausea and vomiting or in patients with liver disease in whom ammonium chloride is contraindicated [23].

Sodium-Dependent Tests of Distal H$^+$ Secretion

Sodium sulfate or a loop diuretic can be useful to assess Na$^+$-dependent acidification and provide additional mechanistic information to tests based on providing an acidemic stimulus. These agents are used to enhance the negative trans-epithelial voltage in the collecting tubule and therefore the capacity not only for H$^+$ secretion but also K$^+$ secretion [24–27]. Amiloride, by contrast, blocks the collecting tubule Na$^+$ channel and can be used to examine H$^+$ secretion when the trans-epithelial voltage is acutely obliterated [25].

Sodium Sulfate

Normal subjects can lower urine pH maximally after sodium sulfate administration even in the absence of metabolic acidosis, provided that distal Na$^+$ delivery is increased acutely and while collecting tubule avidity for Na$^+$ reabsorption is concurrently stimulated [27]. The latter requirement can be achieved by administration of mineralocorticoid or by placing the subject on a low-Na$^+$ diet (i.e., 20 mEq daily) for 3 days, which stimulates aldosterone release [27]. Aldosterone, in turn, enhances distal Na$^+$ reabsorption. The sodium sulfate infusion test can therefore be performed following the administration of fludrocortisone (1 mg orally over the 12 h preceding the sodium sulfate infusion) or after a few days on a low salt diet [12, 27].

When properly performed, the sodium sulfate test results in a fall in urine pH to below 5.5 (usually below 5.0) [12, 27]. Some subjects may exhibit a late response, so urine collections should continue 2–3 h after the infusion is discontinued. Patients with advanced chronic kidney disease also respond normally to sodium sulfate in terms of lowering urine pH [27]. The increase in acid excretion following sodium sulfate infusion is mainly in the form of NH$_4^+$. The K$^+$ excretory (kaliuretic) response with sodium sulfate administration is also useful in assessing distal K$^+$ secretory capacity. Patients with hyperkalemic distal RTA have subnormal K$^+$ excretion whereas in those with normokalemic distal RTA, K$^+$ excretion increases markedly after sodium sulfate [12, 24–26].

Furosemide Test

Loop diuretics increase collecting duct Na^+ delivery by inhibiting NaCl reabsorption in the loop of Henle. Part of the increase in the load of Na^+ delivered to the distal nephron is reabsorbed in the cortical collecting tubule, creating a favorable trans-epithelial voltage gradient for H^+ and K^+ secretion [24]. This interpretation is supported by the finding that the fall in urine pH and the increase in K^+ excretion caused by furosemide are obliterated by amiloride, an agent that blocks the Na^+ channel in the cortical collecting tubule (CCT) (Fig. 5.3) [24]. The kaliuretic effect of furosemide is also attenuated by amiloride [24].

The difference in K^+ excretion that is seen, at comparable urine flow rates, when furosemide is given alone and when combined with amiloride demonstrates the significant contribution of the amiloride-sensitive (i.e., Na^+-dependent) component of distal K^+ secretion [24].

The furosemide test is performed by first collecting a urine sample and then giving 40–80 mg of furosemide orally [24]. Urine pH measured 2–4 h following furosemide should be below 5.5. The test was originally described without prior administration of mineralocorticoid or prior salt restriction to enhance Na^+ avidity [24]. All subjects responded consistently by lowering urine pH below 5.5 without prior use of these maneuvers to enhance avidity distal Na^+ reabsorption. More recent studies have used the furosemide test following administration of mineralocorticoid [28]. While this ensures that distal Na^+ reabsorption is stimulated we think the furosemide test is reliable usually even without preexisting mineralocorticoid administration [24]. Furosemide when given intravenously [29] or bumetanide administration orally [25] have also been shown to lower urine pH consistently.

Amiloride Test

The amiloride test is performed by giving 20 mg of amiloride orally after a baseline urine collection followed by hourly urine collections for measurement of urine pH and electrolyte excretion [25]. Amiloride at low doses blocks apical Na^+ channels in the cortical collecting duct [25]. Administration of amiloride predictably increases urine pH and decreases urine K^+ excretion in normal individuals [25]. In patients with a hyperkalemic DRTA due to a presumed voltage-dependent defect, amiloride should not lead to a normal increase in urine pH or a further decrease in K^+ excretion. A normal response to amiloride (i.e., an increase in urine pH and a decrease in K^+ secretion) implies that voltage-dependent H^+ and K^+ secretion is essentially intact [25].

Fig. 5.3 The effect of furosemide (*filled circle*) and furosemide + amiloride (*open circle*) on urinary acidification in normal subjects. Please note that the lowering effect of furosemide is prevented when amiloride is given concurrently indicating that the effect takes place in the cortical collecting tubule. The *asterisk* denotes a significant difference between the two experimental conditions. Modified from Batlle DC. Segmental characterization of defects in collecting tubule acidification. Kidney Int 1986;30:546–54

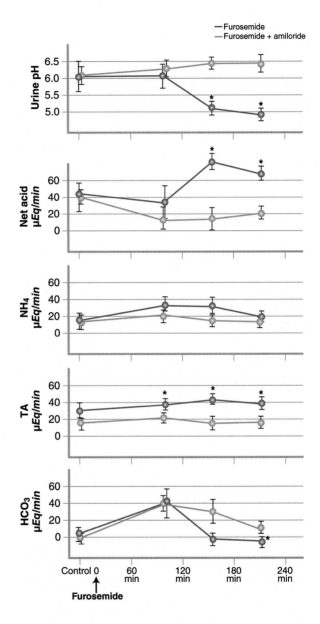

Urinary PCO₂ as an Index of Collecting Tubule H Secretion

Another test to evaluate distal H⁺ ion secretion is assessment of urine PCO_2 in a highly alkaline urine [30, 31]. Sodium HCO_3^- is given, usually intravenously, to increase urine HCO_3^- concentration to a very high values (urine pH approximately

7.8) [31]. This leads to a rise in urine PCO_2 to values considerably higher than blood PCO_2 [31, 32]. Normal subjects achieve values of urine PCO_2 higher than 80 mmHg whereas patients with defects in distal acidification typically fail to increase urine PCO_2 above 60 mmHg [31, 32]. This test, although cumbersome to execute, is a sensitive test of maximal capacity for collecting tubule H^+ ion secretion. A subnormal rise in urine PCO_2, for example, reflects the presence of an "incomplete" type of distal RTA [31, 33].

All patients with distal RTA are expected to have subnormal values of urine PCO_2 after sodium bicarbonate loading, with the exception of distal RTA secondary to Amphotericin B. In amphotericin induced distal RTA, distal H^+ secretion is intact; the acidification defect is due to back leak of H^+ normally secreted. After bicarbonate loading urine is so alkaline that luminal H^+ concentration is reduced and therefore the back leak of H^+ is attenuated. Another situation where urine PCO_2 could theoretically increase normally is distal RTA due to mistargeting of the Cl^-/HCO_3^- exchanger to the apical membrane. HCO_3^- secretion would be increased in this theoretical type of DRTA causing urine PCO_2 to increase despite an alteration in the Cl^-/HCO_3^- exchanger that reduces net distal acidification. In all other types of distal RTA, a subnormal urine PCO_2 is expected, reflecting that the rate of distal H^+ secretion is decreased.

Another tool to evaluate distal H^+ ion secretion is assessment of urine PCO_2 after the infusion of neutral sodium phosphate [34, 35]. Urine PCO_2 is critically dependent on urine phosphate concentration when the pH of the urine is close to 6.8, the pK of the phosphate buffer system. Under these conditions, phosphate rather than HCO_3^- is responsible for generating CO_2 in the urine. By contrast, in the highly alkaline urine (pH > 7.8) produced by sodium bicarbonate loading, phosphate plays no role in the generation of urine PCO_2. This test is performed by infusing neutral phosphate (1 mmol/L total body water in 180 cm^3 of normal saline) slowly at a rate of 1 mL/min for 3 h. Urine phosphate concentration must increase to about 20 mmol/L in two or three successive urine collections after the beginning of the phosphate infusion. Under these conditions, distal H^+ secretion is stimulated and urine PCO_2 rises consistently above 80 mmHg both in normal subjects and in patients with advanced CKD. This usually results in at least twofold increase in plasma phosphate concentration and this makes this test problematic. A similar increase in urine PCO_2 has been reported using oral phosphate loading which may be more practical.

The provocative tests of distal acidification above described are not commonly used and clearly are not needed for clinical diagnosis. The oral furosemide test, however, is easy to perform at bedside or in an outpatient clinical setting and has a role in the evaluation of individuals suspected of having defects in distal acidification. The 3-day NH_4Cl test remains the traditional test in the evaluation of individuals suspected of DRTA. Individuals with kidney stones, osteoporosis, or relatives of individuals with some types of hereditary DRTA may be occasionally diagnosed of incomplete DRTA if they fail to lower urine pH below using this test. However, the definition of incomplete DRTA should include further evidence of impaired distal H^+ secretion.

References

1. Coe FL, Parks JH. The kidney: physiology and pathophysiology. In: Seldin DW, Giebisch G, editors. Pathogenesis and treatment of nephrolithiasis. Philadelphia: Lippincott Williams & Wilkins; 2000. p. 1841–67.
2. Batlle D, Chen S, Haque SK. Physiologic principles in the clinical evaluation of electrolyte, water, and acid–base disorders. In: Seldin DW, Giebisch G, editors. The kidney: physiology and pathophysiology. 5th ed. New York: Raven Press; 2012.
3. Yi JH, Shin HJ, Kim SM, Han SW, Kim HJ, Oh MS. Does the exposure of urine samples to air affect diagnostic tests for urine acidification? Clin J Am Soc Nephrol. 2012;7(8):1211–6.
4. Rodriguez JS, et al. Proximal renal tubular acidosis. A defect in bicarbonate reabsorption with normal urinary acidification. Pediatr Res. 1967;1(2):81–98.
5. Haque SK, Ariceta G, Batlle D. Proximal renal tubular acidosis: a not so rare disorder of multiple etiologies. Nephrol Dial Transplant. 2012;27(12):4273–87.
6. Batlle DC, von Riotte A, Schlueter W. Urinary sodium in the evaluation of hyperchloremic metabolic acidosis. N Engl J Med. 1987;316(3):140–4.
7. Batlle D, Haque SK. Genetic causes and mechanisms of distal renal tubular acidosis. Nephrol Dial Transplant. 2012;27:3691–704.
8. Maalouf NM, Cameron MA, Moe OW, Sakhaee K. Metabolic basis for low urine pH in type 2 diabetes. Clin J Am Soc Nephrol. 2010;5(7):1277–81.
9. Goorno WE, Rector Jr FC, Seldin DW. Relation of renal gluconeogenesis to ammonia production in the dog and rat. Am J Physiol. 1967;213(4):969–74.
10. Mitra A, Batlle D. Acid–base and electrolytes disorders. In: Aldosterone deficiency and resistance. Philadelphia: Saunders; 2002. p. 413–33.
11. Batlle DC. Sodium-dependent urinary acidification in patients with aldosterone deficiency and in adrenalectomized rats: effect of furosemide. Metabolism. 1986;35(9):852–60.
12. Batlle DC, Arruda JA, Kurtzman NA. Hyperkalemic distal renal tubular acidosis associated with obstructive uropathy. N Engl J Med. 1981;304(7):373–80.
13. Crawford MA, Milne MD, Scribner BH. The effects of changes in acid–base balance on urinary citrate in the rat. J Physiol. 1959;149:413–23.
14. Batlle DC, Itsarayoungyuen K, Downer M, Foley R, Arruda J, Kurtzman N, 1983. Suppression of distal urinary acidification after recovery from chronic hypocapnia. Am J Physiol 1983;245(4):F433–42.
15. Batlle DC, Hizon M, Cohen E, Gutterman C, Gupta R. The use of the urinary anion gap in the diagnosis of hyperchloremic metabolic acidosis. N Engl J Med. 1988;318(10):594–9.
16. Adrogue H, Nicolaos M. Tools for clinical assessment. In: Acid–base disorders and their treatment. London: Taylor & Francis Group; 2005. p. 801–48.
17. Nash MA, Torrado AD, Greifer I, Spitzer A, Edelmann Jr CM. Renal tubular acidosis in infants and children. Clinical course, response to treatment, and prognosis. J Pediatr. 1972;80(5):738–48.
18. Lemann Jr J, Adams ND, Wilz DR, Brenes LG. Acid and mineral balances and bone in familial proximal renal tubular acidosis. Kidney Int. 2000;58(3):1267–77.
19. Brenes LG, Sanchez MI. Impaired urinary ammonium excretion in patients with isolated proximal renal tubular acidosis. J Am Soc Nephrol. 1993;4(4):1073–8.
20. Ahya SN, Soler MJ, Levitsky J, Batlle D. Acid–base and potassium disorders in liver disease. Semin Nephrol. 2006;26(6):466–70.
21. Gauthier P, Simon EE, Lemann J. Acid–base and electrolyte disorder in acidosis of chronic renal failure. Philadelphia: Suanders; 2002. p. 207–16.
22. Batlle DC, Sabatini S, Kurzman N. On the mechanism of toluene-induced renal tubular acidosis. Nephron. 1988;49:210–8.
23. Moorthi K, Batlle D. Renal tubular acidosis. In: Gennari FJ, Adrogue HJ, Galla JH, Madias NE, editors. Acid–base disorders and their treatment. Boca Raton: Taylor & Francis Group; 2005. p. 417–67.

24. Batlle DC. Segmental characterization of defects in collecting tubule acidification. Kidney Int. 1986;30(4):546–54.
25. Schlueter W, Keilani T, Hizon M, Kaplan B, Batlle DC. On the mechanism of impaired distal acidification in hyperkalemic renal tubular acidosis: evaluation with amiloride and bumetanide. J Am Soc Nephrol. 1992;3(4):953–64.
26. Batlle DC. Hyperkalemic hyperchloremic metabolic acidosis associated with selective aldosterone deficiency and distal renal tubular acidosis. Semin Nephrol. 1981;1:260–74.
27. Schwartz WB, Jenson RL, Relman AS. Acidification of the urine and increased ammonium excretion without change in acid–base equilibrium: sodium reabsorption as a stimulus to the acidifying process. J Clin Invest. 1955;34(5):673–80.
28. Walsh SB, Shirley DG, Wrong OM, Unwin RJ. Urinary acidification assessed by simultaneous furosemide and fludrocortisone treatment: an alternative to ammonium chloride. Kidney Int. 2007;71(12):1310–6.
29. Rastogi S, Bayliss JM, Nascimento L, Arruda JA. Hyperkalemic renal tubular acidosis: effect of furosemide in humans and in rats. Kidney Int. 1985;28(5):801–7.
30. Halperin ML, Goldstein MB, Haig A, Johnson MD, Stinebaugh BJ. Studies on the pathogenesis of type I (distal) renal tubular acidosis as revealed by the urinary PCO_2 tensions. J Clin Invest. 1974;53(3):669–77.
31. Batlle D, Gaviria M, Grupp M, Arruda JA, Wynn J, Kurtzman NA. Distal nephron function in patients receiving chronic lithium therapy. Kidney Int. 1982;21(3):477–85.
32. Donckerwolcke RA, Valk C, van Wijngaarden-Penterman MJ, van Stekelenburg GJ. The diagnostic value of the urine to blood carbon dioxide tension gradient for the assessment of distal tubular hydrogen secretion in pediatric patients with renal tubular disorders. Clin Nephrol. 1983;19(5):254–8.
33. Batlle DC, Grupp M, Gaviria M. Distal renal tubular acidosis with intact capacity to lower urinary pH. Am J Med. 1982;72:751–8.
34. Batlle DC, Sehy JT, Roseman MK, et al. Clinical and pathophysiologic spectrum of acquired distal renal tubular acidosis. Kidney Int. 1981;20:389–96.
35. Stinebaugh BJ, Scholoeder FX, Gharafry E, et al. Mechanism by which neutral phosphate infusion elevates urine PCO_2. J Lab Clin Med. 1977;89:946–58.

Chapter 6
Pathophysiologic Approach to Metabolic Acidosis

Nitin Relia and Daniel Batlle

Introduction

Metabolic acidosis is a process whereby (1) an excess nonvolatile acid load is placed on the body due to excess acid generation or diminished acid removal by normal homeostatic mechanisms; or (2) bicarbonate is lost from the body [1–4]. While metabolic acidosis is usually suspected when plasma bicarbonate is reduced, the clinician must be aware that metabolic acidosis might be present in a patient with normal or even increased plasma bicarbonate if the metabolic acidosis is part of a mixed acid–base disorder. In addition, subclinical metabolic acidosis can occur when plasma bicarbonate is normal or minimally reduced. This type of metabolic acidosis is known as eubicarbonatemic metabolic acidosis [1]. It can be viewed as a subclinical form of acidosis that nonetheless has potential morbidity in terms of disturbed bone and/or protein metabolism and possibly enhances progression of chronic kidney disease (CKD).

Plasma Chloride and the Plasma Anion Gap

The presence or absence of hyperchloremia is useful in the evaluation of metabolic acidosis. When plasma chloride is increased and plasma sodium normal, either a chronic respiratory alkalosis or a hyperchloremic metabolic acidosis is present [2]. An arterial blood gas is usually needed to distinguish with certainty between a metabolic acidosis and a chronic respiratory alkalosis. The clinical setting coupled with

N. Relia, M.D. (✉) • D. Batlle, M.D.
Division of Nephrology and Hypertension, Northwestern University Feinberg School of Medicine, 320 E. Superior, Chicago, IL 60611, USA
e-mail: docnrelia@gmail.com; d-batlle@northwestern.edu

© Springer Science+Business Media New York 2016
D.E. Wesson (ed.), *Metabolic Acidosis*, DOI 10.1007/978-1-4939-3463-8_6

the use of urinary anion gap (UAG) is often sufficient for the proper diagnosis while avoiding the invasive blood gas measurement [3]. Calculation of the plasma anion gap and evaluation of urinary acid excretion complete the evaluation of metabolic acidosis. The specific types of high and normal anion gap acidosis are discussed in detail elsewhere in this book.

The type of metabolic acidosis present can be initially approached by assessing whether plasma anion gap (AG) is normal or elevated and helps differentiate hyperchloremic metabolic acidosis (normal AG) from high AG metabolic acidosis. Although these categories can overlap the classification is nevertheless very useful to clinicians [3–5]. In a pure hyperchloremic metabolic acidosis, there is an increase in plasma chloride equivalent to the fall in plasma bicarbonate, so that the sum of these two anions remains unchanged [1–3, 5]. An increase in plasma chloride proportional to an increase in plasma sodium usually reflects dehydration. In this case plasma anion gap does not change appreciably [2, 3].

A clinical setting in which the AG may be misleadingly low is hypoalbuminemic states [6–8]. Albumin is negatively charged and makes up a significant portion of unmeasured anions [7]. Therefore, hypoalbuminemia will lead to an underestimation of the size of the AG and potentially to a failure to recognize a clinically important high AG metabolic acidosis. To circumvent this issue, the effect of serum albumin on the plasma AG must be taken into account in the analysis of acid–base disturbances. Figge et al. derived a formula for the plasma AG that takes into account serum albumin, which is based on a mathematical model that has been verified by experiments in vitro [6]. This formula is as follows:

$$\text{Albumin-corrected AG} = \text{AG} + 2.5 \times (4.4 - \text{albumin in g} / \text{dl})$$

For each 1-g/dl decrease in serum albumin below 4.4 g/dl, the observed AG underestimates the actual concentration of unmeasured anions by about 2.5 mEq/l. This estimation has been shown to correlate more or less with other formulas that take into account the effect of plasma albumin on the anion gap [3, 7]. An alternative would be to simply accept that hypoalbuminemia leads to a low anion gap and to use this "baseline" anion gap as the basis for comparison with the observed anion gap in an acid–base disorder. For example, if a patient with nephrotic syndrome chronically has an albumin of 2.5 g/dl and the anion gap is typically low around 7 mEq/l, then a current anion gap of 12, though seemingly normal, would constitute an elevated anion gap of 5 units for this patient and should trigger a search for the cause [3].

A low plasma AG is seen in certain IgG myelomas in which the cationic nature of the paraprotein causes a rise in chloride anions in order to balance the protein's cationic charge [8]. In contrast, the plasma anion gap is normal or even increased in multiple myeloma associated with IgA and IgG paraproteins [8]. IgG paraproteins have isoelectric points that are higher than physiologic pH and are positively charged. The converse takes place with IgA paraproteins, which have isoelectric points below physiologic pH. They behave like anions and when present in large concentrations, the anion gap should increase. In IgA myeloma, however, the AG is usually normal as a result of co-existing hypoalbuminemia, which may reduce an otherwise elevated AG to a normal level. Thus, the interpretation of the plasma AG requires a careful review of all the possible variables that may affect it [3].

An additional limitation with the use of plasma AG occurs in the detection of mixed metabolic acid–base disturbances [9]. The relationship between the increase in the anion gap above normal (ΔAG) and the decrease in serum bicarbonate concentration below normal (ΔHCO_3^-) helps uncover the presence of a mixed acid–base disorders (typically a high AG metabolic acidosis accompanied by either a metabolic alkalosis or a normal AG metabolic acidosis).

Deviations from the presumed 1:1 ratio in this relationship (ΔAG/ΔHCO_3^-) that is present in a high AG metabolic acidosis have been used to diagnose these complex acid–base disturbances [6, 9]. When the ΔHCO_3^- (using a mean normal value for bicarbonate of 24 mEq/l) exceeds the ΔAG, a normal AG metabolic acidosis co-exists. Conversely, when the ΔAG exceeds the ΔHCO_3^-, a metabolic alkalosis is present in addition to the high AG metabolic acidosis. Several studies, however, have indicated that there is variability in this ratio, such that a deviation from a 1:1 ratio may not necessarily indicate the presence of a co-existing normal AG acidosis or metabolic alkalosis. This is due to the fact that this 1:1 ratio may be transient and/ or dependent on the type of metabolic acidosis present [6, 8, 10–12]. Studies involving ketoacidosis or lactic acidosis, as well as rarer causes of organic acid accumulation such as toluene poisoning, showed that ratios either greater than 1 or less than 0.8 (the latter being less common) were observed in the absence of an apparent co-existing metabolic alkalosis or normal AG acidosis [8, 10, 13–18]. This underscores the importance of considering patient history, physical examination, or other laboratory data in accurately defining an acid–base disorder. Nonetheless, the plasma AG, with all the previously mentioned caveats, provides a convenient "starting point" in the evaluation of metabolic acidosis and helps to monitor over time the presumed changes in unmeasured anions responsible for the anion gap such as lactate during therapy for metabolic acidosis in the acute setting.

Acid Excretion by the Kidney in Metabolic Acidosis

Two major components of acid excretion are stimulated as part of the homeostatic response to chronic metabolic acidosis: excretion of acids collectively referred to as "titratable acids" and excretion of ammonium. Excretion of both leads to the formation of "new" bicarbonate [3]. In addition, bicarbonate is also formed from the metabolism of retained organic anions such as citrate which represents potential alkali [19].

Titratable Acids

Metabolic acidosis typically increases acid excretion which prevents further and sustained acidosis and contributes to recovery from this acid–base disorder. Titratable acids are urine solutes that buffer secreted protons (H^+), enabling H^+

excretion without substantial decreases in urine pH (or equivalently, increases in urine free H^+ concentration) [20]. Multiple solutes such as phosphoric acid, sulfuric acid, and creatinine contribute to what is collectively referred to as titratable acid excretion. Phosphate is the predominant component, typically accounting for more than 50 % of total titratable acid [20, 21]. At a typical serum pH of 7.4, approximately 80 % of filtered phosphate is HPO_4^{2-} and 20 % is $H_2PO_4^-$.

Titratable acid excretion in the form of phosphate reflects the amount of filtered HPO_4^{2-} that buffers H^+ secreted in the proximal tubule, loop of Henle, distal tubule, and collecting duct. The proximal tubule is the primary site of phosphate reabsorption and is the nephron location where metabolic acidosis and other acid–base disorders regulate phosphate transport [19]. Acute and chronic metabolic acidosis decrease proximal tubule phosphate reabsorption through a variety of mechanisms including decreased apical plasma membrane Na^+-dependent phosphate transport [22, 23]. Metabolic acidosis decreases luminal pH as a result of decreased filtered bicarbonate load and increased H^+ secretion. Luminal acidification then independently inhibits proximal tubule phosphate uptake causing phosphaturia [24, 25]. Metabolic acidosis also increases PTH release and PTH inhibits proximal tubule phosphate reabsorption, increasing luminal phosphate availability as a titratable acid and thereby promoting urine net acid excretion in response to metabolic acidosis. The effect of metabolic acidosis on FGF 23, another potent phosphaturic hormone, is unclear. A reduction in plasma FGF 23 levels has been reported during chronic metabolic acidosis [26]. This somewhat unexpected finding would lead to decrease in phosphate in urine and less titratable acid excretion. Further research in this area will help clarify the role of FGF 23 with respect to titratable acid excretion.

Acidosis-induced changes in phosphate excretion depend on systemic phosphate availability. When dietary phosphate is restricted, basal phosphate excretion is greatly reduced and the typical increase in urinary phosphate excretion in response to metabolic acidosis is greatly blunted [27]. Changes in extra kidney phosphate metabolism could contribute to increased phosphate availability for excretion as titratable acid. Metabolic acidosis increases small intestine Na^+-dependent phosphate uptake and this is associated with increased expression of both protein and mRNA for the primary small intestinal apical plasma membrane phosphate transporter NaPi-IIb [28]. There is also increased phosphate release from bone in response to both acute and chronic metabolic acidosis [29]. The net effect of these extra kidney effects is to enable changes in urinary phosphate excretion for buffering protons without causing a change in systemic phosphate concentration in response to changes in systemic acid–base status. Nevertheless, the ability to enhance net acid excretion by increasing phosphate and thus titratable acidity is limited. Importantly, increased NH_4^+ excretion provides the major adaptive increase in net acid excretion in response to a chronic acid challenge to systemic acid–base status.

Ammonium (NH_4^+)

Ammonia is produced by almost all kidney epithelial cells but the proximal tubule is quantitatively the primary site for ammoniagenesis. Glutamine is the primary metabolic substrate for ammoniagenesis. An essential initial adaptive response to metabolic acidosis is increased extraction and catabolism of plasma glutamine that occurs predominately in the proximal convoluted tubule [19]. The resulting increase in kidney ammoniagenesis and NH_4^+ transport into the urine accomplish the final excretion of acid by trapping secreted hydrogen ions with NH_3 and forming NH_4^+. Acute onset of metabolic acidosis produces a rapid and pronounced increase in renal catabolism of glutamine [30]. Within 1–3 h, arterial plasma glutamine concentration increases twofold [31] due to increased release of glutamine from muscle and liver [32]. Uptake of glutamine through the basolateral membrane of proximal tubule cell occurs by reversal of the neutral amino acid exchanger LAT 2 and through increased expression of a basolateral glutamine transporter SNAT3. In addition, the transport of glutamine into the mitochondria may be acutely activated [33]. Acidosis enhances gene expression of enzymes involved in glutamine metabolism and gluconeogenesis that leads to production of ammonium and bicarbonate, respectively. Additional responses include acute activation of NHE3 [34]. This process facilitates rapid removal of cellular NH_4^+ and ensures that the bulk of NH_4^+ generated from the amide and amine nitrogens of glutamine is excreted in the urine [35]. Finally, cellular concentrations of glutamate and α-ketoglutarate are significantly decreased within the rat renal cortex [36]. The latter compounds are products and inhibitors of the glutaminase and glutamate dehydrogenase reactions, respectively. The acute increase in renal ammoniagenesis results from a rapid activation of key transport processes, an increased availability of glutamine, and a decrease in product inhibition of the enzymes of ammoniagenesis. Several transport proteins mediate medullary NH_4^+ reabsorption by the thick ascending loop of Henle [37]. The mechanisms that maintain high interstitial NH_4^+ concentrations in the medulla and papilla, thereby limiting NH_4^+ backflux into the systemic circulation, remain elusive. A role of sulfatides in kidney NH_4^+ handling, urinary acidification, and acid–base homeostasis has been recently proposed [38]. In mammals, sulfatides accumulate in the kidney with particularly high concentrations in distal nephron segments and the renal medulla [39]. The major renal sulfatide in humans and rodents is the galactosylceramide(GalCer)-derived SM4s. Sulfatides, most probably by their anionic extracellular charge, are required to maintain high interstitial NH_4^+ concentration in the papilla. This high interstitial NH_4^+ concentration is needed for urine NH_4^+ excretion under basal conditions and during metabolic acidosis [38].

The net effect is that NH_4^+ excretion can increase from its basal level of 30–40 mEq/day to more than 200–300 mEq/day with severe and persistent metabolic acidosis [40–42]. This marked ability to increase in NH_4^+ excretion contrasts with the more limited ability to increase titratable acid by increasing phosphate excretion due to lack of an increase in plasma phosphate levels with attendant increased phosphaturia.

Citrate

Citrate is an organic anion and serves a dual purpose in the urine. For humans ingesting Western diets that are typically acid-producing, urine in their basal state has a negligible amount of HCO_3^- whereas citrate is the main urine base under these basal conditions (~500 mg/day) [19]. In addition to base excretion, the 1:1 Ca^{2+}:Citrate^{3-} complex has a very high association constant and solubility. These properties make citrate the most effective Ca^{2+} chelator in the urine under basal conditions, thereby preventing Ca^{2+} precipitation with phosphate and oxalate [43, 44]. Consequently, low urine citrate excretion (hypocitraturia) is a major underlying cause of human kidney stones [43].

Urine citrate is in millimolar quantities under basal conditions and regulation of its kidney handling is entirely by the proximal tubule (Fig. 6.1). Reabsorption of filtered citrate occurs in the proximal tubule apical membrane by NaDC1 (SLC13A2), an Na1-dependent dicarboxylic acid co-transporter [45]. Although citrate is in equilibrium between its divalent and trivalent forms in the proximal tubule lumen, its divalent form (citrate^{2-}) is the transported species. Once it is absorbed from the proximal tubule lumen, citrate can be metabolized by cytoplasmic ATP citrate lyase to oxaloacetate and acetyl-CoA or shuttled into the mitochondria to enter the citric acid cycle [46]. When citrate$^{2-/3-}$ is converted to CO_2 and H_2O, 2 or 3 H^+ are consumed. Therefore, each milliequivalent of citrate excreted in the urine is tantamount to 2 or 3 OH^- loss [44].

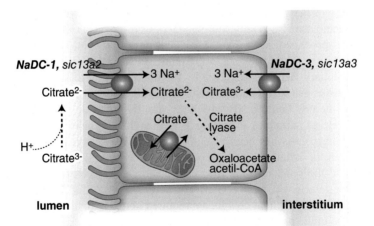

Fig. 6.1 Scheme for the metabolism of citrate in a proximal tubule cell. The carrier NADC-1 of apical membrane reabsorbs the bivalent citrate. In conditions of acidosis the presence of H^+ in the proximal tubule fluid stimulates the formation of citrate bivalent from trivalent. The divalent citrate is reabsorbed and metabolized by citrate lyase or through the tricarboxylic acid cycle in the mitochondria of proximal tubular cells. NADC-1 (SLC13A2)=Na-dependent low affinity carrier of dicarboxylic acids. NADC-3 (SLC13A3)=Na-dependent high affinity carrier of dicarboxylic acids. Modified from Dogliotti et al. *Journal of Translational Medicine* 2013 11:109. doi:10.1186/1479-5876-11-109

With metabolic acidosis there is an adaptative increase in citrate uptake and metabolism within the proximal tubule, reducing urine base excretion. In this way citrate retention provides a compensatory mechanism for metabolic acidosis. This adaptive increase in citrate reabsorption occurs by multiple mechanisms [19]. Acidification of lumen pH titrates citrate^{3-} to citrate^{2-}, the latter being the preferred substrate for transport across the proximal tubule as discussed. In addition, low pH directly activates NaDC1 to increase transport independent of divalent citrate [47, 48]. In addition to enhanced citrate transport, increased cellular metabolism also drives citrate reabsorption. After cellular uptake, citrate is metabolized through one of two pathways: a cytoplasmic pathway involving citrate lyase or a mitochondrial pathway involving the citric acid cycle [46] (Fig. 6.1).

During metabolic acidosis, the cytoplasmic citrate lyase and mitochondrial aconitase activities also increase [49]. Because both pathways generate HCO_3^-, increased citrate reabsorption is equivalent to a decreased base excretion that leads to decreased urine citrate concentration and pH, the latter being a tubular milieu favoring kidney stone formation [19, 50]. Consequently, this adaptive response to mitigate metabolic acidosis comes at the cost of increased risk for kidney stones and helps explain the increased stone risk in states characterized by chronic metabolic acidosis such as renal tubular acidosis [51, 52].

Net Acid Excretion

The traditional formula for net acid excretion is as follows:

$$\text{Net acid excretion} = U_{NH_4^+} + U_{\text{Titratable acid}} - U_{HCO_3^-}$$

To more comprehensively describe the kidney role in acid–base balance using the urine net acid excretion formula, it is necessary to include the portion of daily dietary alkali load that is excreted in the form of organic anions which can be metabolized to HCO_3^-. Thus, urine excretion of organic anions represents loss of potential HCO_3^- [53]. A formula for net acid excretion that would take this into account is as follows:

$$\text{Revised net acid excretion} = (U_{NH_4^+} + U_{\text{Titrated acid}}) - (U_{HCO_3^-} + U_{\text{Potential HCO}_3^-})$$

In normal subjects urine pH is approximately 6.0 for the majority of measurements performed during a 24-h period [54]. This suggests that the urine contains little HCO_3^- and therefore $U_{HCO_3^-}$ can be considered negligible at this urine pH. Rather than increasing HCO_3^- excretion, dietary alkali is converted initially to HCO_3^- in the liver and is then titrated through the production of organic acids such as citrate. Under normal conditions, approximately 40 % of NAE is in the form of TA and 60 % is in the form of ammonia; urine HCO_3^- is essentially zero and urinary organic anions such as citrate represent the main mode of base excretion. During metabolic acidosis and with chronic acid loads there is also a decrease in the base excretion such as citrate and other organic anions [55, 56]. It should therefore be noted that a low level of citrate excretion may be a clue to the presence of subclinical or eubicarbonatemic metabolic acidosis. Since urine HCO_3^- is typically low under most basal conditions, low urine citrate might better reflect adaptation to subtle metabolic acidosis than urine HCO_3^-. Ideally, all components of net acid excretion should be part of the evaluation of metabolic acidosis.

Implications for Alkali Therapy

Traditionally, alkali therapy has been reserved for patients with acute or chronic metabolic acidosis. The primary purpose in treating chronic metabolic acidosis associated with CKD has been to prevent morbidities related to bone disease, improve the nutritional status, and prevent muscle protein breakdown [1–4, 57]. These goals are themselves very good reasons to use alkali therapy in the CKD population with chronic metabolic acidosis. Data from animal and observational studies in patients with non-dialysis dependent CKD also suggest that lower serum HCO_3^- concentrations are associated with a higher risk of progressive kidney function loss [58–60]. Additionally, data from non-dialysis CKD patients has shown association of higher HCO_3^- levels (>22–24 mmol/l) with lower mortality and improved kidney and overall survival outcomes [60–62]. The reason for the association between metabolic acidosis and more rapid progression of CKD is not clear but it seems logical to postulate that the need to excrete the daily dietary acid load in CKD promotes an adaptive increase in NH_4^+ excreted per nephron. This may be associated with activation of the complement system, the renin–angiotensin system, and with increased renal production of endothelin-1, all of which may produce tubulointerstitial inflammation and chronic kidney damage [63, 64]. Small randomized trials have hence been conducted and have shown benefits of alkali therapy on slowing CKD progression [61–64]. Dietary acid reduction and alkali-based diets of fruits and vegetables also hold promise as a kidney-protective strategy in CKD management [64].

These recent findings will hopefully foster more research on the potential of alkali-based therapies, the optimal dose, and the time of initiation in the management of the various stages of CKD [65]. Clearly, proper attention to metabolic acidosis and its recognition even in subclinical stages offer opportunities for therapeutic intervention for CKD.

References

1. Alpern RJ, Sakhaee K. The clinical spectrum of chronic metabolic acidosis: homeostatic mechanisms produce significant morbidity. Am J Kidney Dis. 1997;29(2):291–302.
2. Batlle D. Hyperchloremic metabolic acidosis. In: Seldin D, Giebisch G, editors. The regulation of acid–base balance. New York: Raven; 1989. p. 319–51.

3. Batlle D, Chen S, Haque SK. Physiologic principles in the clinical evaluation of electrolyte, water, and acid–base disorders. In: Seldin DW, Giebisch G, editors. The kidney: physiology and pathophysiology. 5th ed. New York: Raven; 2012.
4. Kraut JA, Madias NE. Metabolic acidosis: pathophysiology, diagnosis and management. Nat Rev Nephrol. 2010;6(5):274–85.
5. Oh MS, Carroll HJ. The anion gap. N Engl J Med. 1977;297(15):814–7.
6. Figge J, Rossing TH, Fencl V. The role of serum proteins in acid–base equilibria. J Lab Clin Med. 1991;117(6):453–67.
7. Feldman M, Soni N, Dickson B. Influence of hypoalbuminemia or hyperalbuminemia on the serum anion gap. J Lab Clin Med. 2005;146(6):317–20.
8. De Troyer A, Stolarczyk A, De Beyl DZ, Stryckmans P. Value of anion-gap determination in multiple myeloma. N Engl J Med. 1977;296(15):858–60.
9. Narins RG, Emmett M. Simple and mixed acid–base disorders: a practical approach. Medicine (Baltimore). 1980;59(3):161–87.
10. Adrogue HJ, Wilson H, Boyd 3rd AE, Suki WN, Eknoyan G. Plasma acid–base patterns in diabetic ketoacidosis. N Engl J Med. 1982;307(26):1603–10.
11. Orringer CE, Eustace JC, Wunsch CD, Gardner LB. Natural history of lactic acidosis after grand-mal seizures. A model for the study of an anion-gap acidosis not associated with hyperkalemia. N Engl J Med. 1977;297(15):796–9.
12. Paulson WD. Anion gap-bicarbonate relation in diabetic ketoacidosis. Am J Med. 1986;81(6):995–1000.
13. Uribarri J, Oh MS, Carroll HJ. D-Lactic acidosis. A review of clinical presentation, biochemical features, and pathophysiologic mechanisms. Medicine (Baltimore). 1998;77(2):73–82.
14. Adrogue HJ, Eknoyan G, Suki WK. Diabetic ketoacidosis: role of the kidney in the acid–base homeostasis re-evaluated. Kidney Int. 1984;25(4):591–8.
15. Brivet F, Bernardin M, Cherin P, Chalas J, Galanaud P, Dormont J. Hyperchloremic acidosis during grand mal seizure lactic acidosis. Intensive Care Med. 1994;20(1):27–31.
16. Carlisle EJ, Donnelly SM, Vasuvattakul S, Kamel KS, Tobe S, Halperin ML. Glue-sniffing and distal renal tubular acidosis: sticking to the facts. J Am Soc Nephrol. 1991;1(8):1019–27.
17. Oh MS, Carroll HJ, Uribarri J. Mechanism of normochloremic and hyperchloremic acidosis in diabetic ketoacidosis. Nephron. 1990;54(1):1–6.
18. Oster JR, Singer I, Contreras GN, Ahmad HI, Vieira CF. Metabolic acidosis with extreme elevation of anion gap: case report and literature review. Am J Med Sci. 1999;317(1):38–49.
19. Curthoys NP, Moe OW. Proximal tubule function and response to acidosis. Clin J Am Soc Nephrol. 2014;9(9):1627–38.
20. Hamm LL, Simon EE. Roles and mechanisms of urinary buffer excretion. Am J Physiol. 1987;253(4 Pt 2):F595–605.
21. Wrong O, Davies HE. The excretion of acid in renal disease. Q J Med. 1959;28(110):259–313.
22. Ambuhl PM, Zajicek HK, Wang H, Puttaparthi K, Levi M. Regulation of renal phosphate transport by acute and chronic metabolic acidosis in the rat. Kidney Int. 1998;53(5):1288–98.
23. Guntupalli J, Eby B, Lau K. Mechanism for the phosphaturia of NH$_4$Cl: dependence on acidemia but not on diet PO$_4$ or PTH. Am J Physiol. 1982;242(5):F552–60.
24. Hoffmann N, Thees M, Kinne R. Phosphate transport by isolated renal brush border vesicles. Pflugers Arch. 1976;362(2):147–56.
25. Ullrich KJ, Rumrich G, Kloss S. Phosphate transport in the proximal convolution of the rat kidney. III. Effect of extracellular and intracellular pH. Pflugers Arch. 1978;377(1):33–42.
26. Domrongkitchaiporn S, Disthabanchong S, Cheawchanthanakij R, Niticharoenpong K, Stitchantrakul W, Charoenphandhu N, Krishnamra N. Oral phosphate supplementation corrects hypophosphatemia and normalizes plasma FGF23 and 25-hydroxyvitamin D3 levels in women with chronic metabolic acidosis. Exp Clin Endocrinol Diabetes. 2010;118(2):105–12.
27. Villa-Bellosta R, Sorribas V. Compensatory regulation of the sodium/phosphate cotransporters NaPi-IIc (SCL34A3) and Pit-2 (SLC20A2) during Pi deprivation and acidosis. Pflugers Arch. 2010;459(3):499–508.

28. Stauber A, Radanovic T, Stange G, Murer H, Wagner CA, Biber J. Regulation of intestinal phosphate transport. II. Metabolic acidosis stimulates Na(+)-dependent phosphate absorption and expression of the Na(+)-P(i) cotransporter NaPi-IIb in small intestine. Am J Physiol Gastrointest Liver Physiol. 2005;288(3):G501–6.

29. Lemann Jr J, Bushinsky DA, Hamm LL. Bone buffering of acid and base in humans. Am J Physiol Renal Physiol. 2003;285(5):F811–32.

30. Tamarappoo BK, Joshi S, Welbourne TC. Interorgan glutamine flow regulation in metabolic acidosis. Miner Electrolyte Metab. 1990;16(5):322–30.

31. Hughey RP, Rankin BB, Curthoys NP. Acute acidosis and renal arteriovenous differences of glutamine in normal and adrenalectomized rats. Am J Physiol. 1980;238(3):F199–204.

32. Schrock H, Cha CJ, Goldstein L. Glutamine release from hindlimb and uptake by kidney in the acutely acidotic rat. Biochem J. 1980;188(2):557–60.

33. Sastrasinh M, Sastrasinh S. Effect of acute pH change on mitochondrial glutamine transport. Am J Physiol. 1990;259(6 Pt 2):F863–6.

34. Horie S, Moe O, Tejedor A, Alpern RJ. Preincubation in acid medium increases Na/H antiporter activity in cultured renal proximal tubule cells. Proc Natl Acad Sci U S A. 1990;87(12):4742–5.

35. Tannen RL, Ross BD. Ammoniagenesis by the isolated perfused rat kidney: the critical role of urinary acidification. Clin Sci (Lond). 1979;56(4):353–64.

36. Lowry M, Ross BD. Activation of oxoglutarate dehydrogenase in the kidney in response to acute acidosis. Biochem J. 1980;190(3):771–80.

37. Weiner ID, Verlander JW. Role of NH3 and NH4+ transporters in renal acid–base transport. Am J Physiol Renal Physiol. 2011;300(1):F11–23.

38. Stettner P, Bourgeois S, Marsching C, Traykova-Brauch M, Porubsky S, Nordstrom V, Hopf C, Koesters R, Sandhoff R, Wiegandt H, Wagner CA, Grone HJ, Jennemann R. Sulfatides are required for renal adaptation to chronic metabolic acidosis. Proc Natl Acad Sci U S A. 2013;110(24):9998–10003.

39. Lullmann-Rauch R, Matzner U, Franken S, Hartmann D, Gieselmann V. Lysosomal sulfoglycolipid storage in the kidneys of mice deficient for arylsulfatase A (ASA) and of double-knockout mice deficient for ASA and galactosylceramide synthase. Histochem Cell Biol. 2001;116(2):161–9.

40. Owen OE, Licht JH, Sapir DG. Renal function and effects of partial rehydration during diabetic ketoacidosis. Diabetes. 1981;30(6):510–8.

41. Clarke E, Evans BM, Macintyre I, Milne MD. Acidosis in experimental electrolyte depletion. Clin Sci (Lond). 1955;14(3):421–40.

42. Goorno WE, Rector Jr FC, Seldin DW. Relation of renal gluconeogenesis to ammonia production in the dog and rat. Am J Physiol. 1967;213(4):969–74.

43. Moe OW. Kidney stones: pathophysiology and medical management. Lancet. 2006;367(9507):333–44.

44. Moe OW, Preisig PA. Dual role of citrate in mammalian urine. Curr Opin Nephrol Hypertens. 2006;15(4):419–24.

45. Pajor AM. Sequence and functional characterization of a renal sodium/dicarboxylate cotransporter. J Biol Chem. 1995;270(11):5779–85.

46. Simpson DP. Citrate excretion: a window on renal metabolism. Am J Physiol. 1983;244(3):F223–34.

47. Brennan S, Hering-Smith K, Hamm LL. Effect of pH on citrate reabsorption in the proximal convoluted tubule. Am J Physiol. 1988;255(2 Pt 2):F301–6.

48. Wright SH, Kippen I, Wright EM. Effect of pH on the transport of Krebs cycle intermediates in renal brush border membranes. Biochim Biophys Acta. 1982;684(2):287–90.

49. Aruga S, Wehrli S, Kaissling B, Moe OW, Preisig PA, Pajor AM, Alpern RJ. Chronic metabolic acidosis increases NaDC-1 mRNA and protein abundance in rat kidney. Kidney Int. 2000;58(1):206–15.

50. Preisig PA. The acid-activated signaling pathway: starting with Pyk2 and ending with increased NHE3 activity. Kidney Int. 2007;72(11):1324–9.

51. Batlle D, Haque SK. Genetic causes and mechanisms of distal renal tubular acidosis. Nephrol Dial Transplant. 2012;27(10):3691–704.
52. Moorthi K, Batlle D. Renal tubular acidosis. In: Gennari FJ, Adrogue HJ, Galla JH, Madias NE, editors. Acid–base disorders and their treatment. Boca Raton: Taylor & Francis Group; 2005. p. 417–67.
53. Halperin ML, Cheema Dhadli S, Kamel KS. Physiology of acid–base balance: links with kidney stone prevention. Semin Nephrol. 2006;26(6):441–6.
54. Coe FL, Parks JH. Pathogenesis and treatment of nephrolithiasis. In: Seldin DW, Giebisch G, editors. The kidney: physiology and pathophysiology. Philadelphia: Lippincott Williams & Wilkins; 2000. p. 1841–67.
55. Crawford MA, Milne MD, Scribner BH. The effects of changes in acid–base balance on urinary citrate in the rat. J Physiol. 1959;149:413–23.
56. Melnick JZ, Preisig PA, Haynes S, Pak CY, Sakhaee K, Alpern RJ. Converting enzyme inhibition causes hypocitraturia independent of acidosis or hypokalemia. Kidney Int. 1998;54(5):1670–4.
57. Mitch WE. Influence of metabolic acidosis on nutrition. Am J Kidney Dis. 1997;29(5):xlvi–xlviii.
58. Raphael KL, Wei G, Baird BC, Greene T, Beddhu S. Higher serum bicarbonate levels within the normal range are associated with better survival and renal outcomes in African Americans. Kidney Int. 2011;79(3):356–62.
59. Shah SN, Abramowitz M, Hostetter TH, Melamed ML. Serum bicarbonate levels and the progression of kidney disease: a cohort study. Am J Kidney Dis. 2009;54(2):270–7.
60. Phisitkul S, Khanna A, Simoni J, Broglio K, Sheather S, Rajab MH, Wesson DE. Amelioration of metabolic acidosis in patients with low GFR reduced kidney endothelin production and kidney injury, and better preserved GFR. Kidney Int. 2010;77(7):617–23.
61. Wesson DE, Simoni J. Increased tissue acid mediates a progressive decline in the glomerular filtration rate of animals with reduced nephron mass. Kidney Int. 2009;75(9):929–35.
62. Sahni V, Rosa RM, Batlle D. Potential benefits of alkali therapy to prevent GFR loss: time for a palatable 'solution' for the management of CKD. Kidney Int. 2010;78(11):1065–7.
63. Mahajan A, Simoni J, Sheather SJ, Broglio KR, Rajab MH, Wesson DE. Daily oral sodium bicarbonate preserves glomerular filtration rate by slowing its decline in early hypertensive nephropathy. Kidney Int. 2010;78(3):303–9.
64. Goraya N, Wesson DE. Dietary management of chronic kidney disease: protein restriction and beyond. Curr Opin Nephrol Hypertens. 2012;21(6):635–40.
65. Kaskel F, Batlle D, Beddhu S, Daugirdas J, Feldman H, Ferris M, Fine L, Freedman BI, Kimmel PL, Flessner MF, Star RA. Kidney Research National Dialogue (KRND). Improving CKD therapies and care: a National Dialogue. Clin J Am Soc Nephrol. 2014;9(4):815–7.

Chapter 7
Dietary Contributions to Metabolic Acidosis

Lynda Frassetto

Case Vignette

A 40 y/o morbidly obese woman comes into your office for a new patient visit. She recently moved to southern Florida after getting a divorce. She has diabetes and high cholesterol levels and takes metformin, lovastatin, and lisinopril. She says her brother, who also has diabetes, high blood pressure, and a history of kidney stones, recently had to stop working because of a stroke that left him paralyzed on his left side. She tells you this has scared her, and now she wants to lose weight and is interested in trying the Atkins diet.

Physical exam reveals that she is 5 feet 5 inches, 225 lbs (BMI 38.6), Caucasian, BP 140/85, with an abdominal girth/hip ratio of 1.3. Her screening labs are unremarkable except for a hemoglobin level of 12.1 g, fasting blood sugar of 120 mg/dL, and total cholesterol of 231 mg/dL. Her thyroid tests are normal. Urine protein to creatinine ratio is 800 mg/g. Should you agree that she can try the Atkins diet for weight loss?

Question

Which one of these BEST explains your response?

A. Yes, the Atkins diet has been shown to help subjects lose weight.
B. No, the Atkins diet is not a good diet for subjects with high blood sugar.

L. Frassetto, M.D. (✉)
Department of Medicine, University of California San Francisco,
505 Parnassus Avenue, Campus Box 0126, Room M1208, San Francisco, CA 94143, USA
e-mail: frassett@gcrc.ucsf.edu

© Springer Science+Business Media New York 2016
D.E. Wesson (ed.), *Metabolic Acidosis*, DOI 10.1007/978-1-4939-3463-8_7

C. Yes, but you should tell her to increase her salt and water intake to help keep herself hydrated.

D. No, the Atkins diet can promote increased acid production and increase her risk for kidney stones.

E. No, the Atkins diet is contraindicated in subjects with high blood lipid levels.

Determinants of Blood pH (Review)

There are at least three independent determinants of the set point for blood hydrogen ion concentration ($[H^+]$): the partial pressure of carbon dioxide (PCO_2), excretion of which is controlled by the lungs [1]; diet acid or base load, including chloride intake from the salt content of the diet [2, 3]; and the kidney, which declines in function with advancing age [4]. In healthy adult humans eating ordinary American diets, these factors help insure that systemic acid–base equilibrium is maintained within narrow limits. This occurs despite the continual addition of acids to the body from cellular metabolism and end products of metabolism of neutral precursors in the diet (Fig. 7.1).

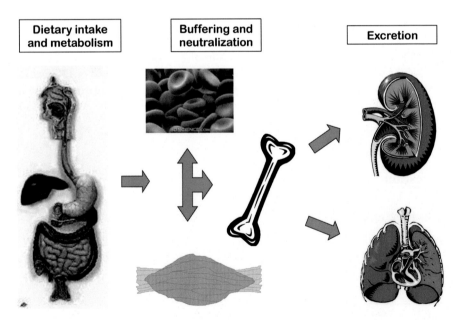

Fig. 7.1 Overview of systemic acid–base balance: intake and metabolism, buffering and neutralization, and excretion

Metabolism of Dietary Substrates

Interest in the effects of food on acid–base balance goes back to the end of the nineteenth century, with studies evaluating the effects of diet on urinary pH and acid excretion [5–7]. In these early studies, subjects would be fed specific diets, and the urine analyzed for compounds such as urea, ammonia, non-urea nitrogen, sulfates, phosphates, and chlorides. Figure 7.2 is a re-analysis of the studies by Blatherwick [7] demonstrating changes in the net quantity of acid (net acid excretion, NAE) excreted by addition of one specific food item to a baseline diet.

Understanding of these processes was furthered by the pioneering group of Relman, Lemann, and Lennon in the late 1950s [8–10]. Studying first liquid and then solid diets, they investigated how renal acid excretion correlated with endogenous acid production, demonstrating that the net acid production was the sum of (1) the oxidation of organic sulfur to sulfates, (2) the net liberation of protons from organic phosphate radicals, and (3) the endogenous formation of unmetabolized organic acids. Some sources of endogenous acids and their metabolism are shown in Fig. 7.3 [11]. Dietary bases come from the ingestion of organic anions such as citrate or malate that are metabolizable to bicarbonate. These investigations culminated in a landmark paper by this group in 1966 [12], demonstrating that the quantity of "fixed" or nonvolatile acids produced from a given diet required knowledge of both the composition of the dietary precursors and the metabolic end products excreted in the urine and feces.[1]

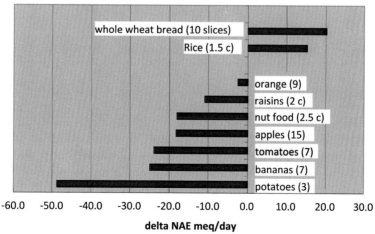

Clinical trial: effect on renal net acid excretion (NAE) of adding one food type to a baseline diet

Fig. 7.2   The effects on renal net acid excretion of adding one food item to a baseline diet [7]

---

[1] Net endogenous acid production=organic acids+sulfates-bicarbonate; Net renal acid excretion=ammonium plus titratable acids minus bicarbonate.

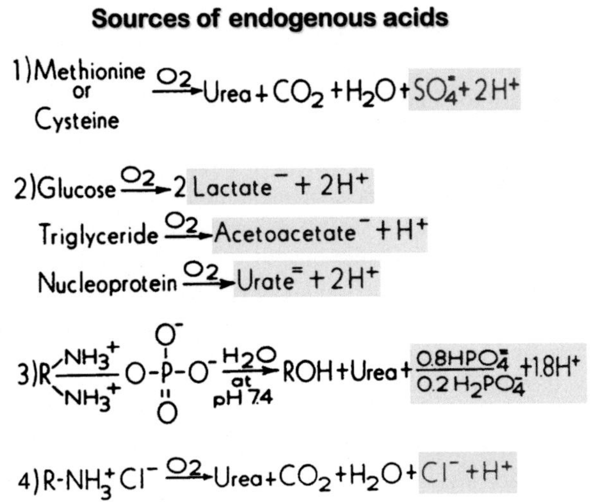

Sources of endogenous acids

$$1)\,\text{Methionine} \atop \text{or} \;\; \text{Cysteine} \xrightarrow{O_2} \text{Urea} + CO_2 + H_2O + SO_4^{=} + 2H^+$$

$$2)\,\text{Glucose} \xrightarrow{O_2} 2\,\text{Lactate}^- + 2H^+$$

$$\text{Triglyceride} \xrightarrow{O_2} \text{Acetoacetate}^- + H^+$$

$$\text{Nucleoprotein} \xrightarrow{O_2} \text{Urate}^= + 2H^+$$

$$3)\,R\!\!\begin{array}{c}{}^{NH_3^+}\\{}_{NH_3^+}\end{array}\!\!O\!-\!\overset{O^-}{\underset{O}{\overset{|}{P}}}\!-\!O^- \xrightarrow[\text{at pH 7.4}]{H_2O} ROH + \text{Urea} + \frac{0.8\,HPO_4^=}{0.2\,H_2PO_4^-} + 1.8H^+$$

$$4)\,R\text{-}NH_3^+\,Cl^- \xrightarrow{O_2} \text{Urea} + CO_2 + H_2O + Cl^- + H^+$$

Fig. 7.3 Dietary sources of endogenous acids [11]

Food analyses show that almost all foods contain acid precursors, while fruits and vegetables also contain base precursors. From these data, formulas for estimating the acid or base dietary effects of various foods have been developed [13–15]. Using dietary estimates avoids having to measure renal NAE, which generally requires a research laboratory. However, use of these formulas requires detailed and quantitative analyses for dietary cations (sodium, potassium, calcium, magnesium) and anions (chloride, sulfate, phosphate). Most of the formulas use an estimate for organic anion production, and some include a factor for intestinal ion absorption.

Effects of Dietary Substrates on Systemic Acid–Base Balance

This foundational work raises a critical question; namely, in healthy subjects with normally functioning kidneys, can changing dietary intake alter systemic acid–base balance, and if so, to what degree? Relman and colleagues concluded that in their healthy subjects, net endogenous acid production was approximately equal to renal NAE. However, re-evaluation of that data by Kurtz et al. [2] (Fig. 7.4) demonstrated that at high acid loads [when endogenous acid production exceeds ~ 1 milliequivalent (mEq)/kg body weight], the normal kidneys cannot excrete all of the metabolic acids produced. Instead, the degree of change in systemic acid–base balance—that is, the levels at which the body maintains the blood pH and bicarbonate—is dependent on the quantity of acid or base consumed. Figure 7.5 demonstrates plasma bicarbonate and renal NAE in healthy older women admitted to a metabolic unit and fed the same high acid load diet for the duration of the study. Addition of either 60 or 120 mEq of oral potassium bicarbonate (KHCO$_3$) for 18 days raised and maintained plasma bicarbonate levels significantly for the duration of the treatment

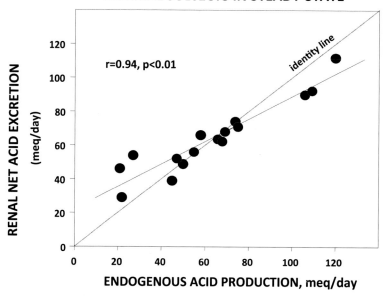

Fig. 7.4 Demonstration that when endogenous acid production $> \sim 1$ mEq/kg, the kidneys are not able to excrete the entire acid load (i.e., RNAE$<$EAP) [2]

Supplementation with oral bicarbonate raises plasma HCO3 levels and lowers renal net acid excretion in a dose-dependent fashion

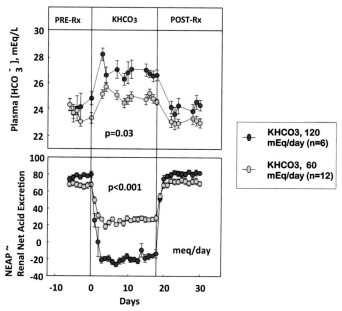

Fig. 7.5 Dose dependent changes in plasma bicarbonate with increasing doses of KHCO₃. Baseline plasma HCO₃ 23.7 ± 1.3, on 60 mEq plasma HCO₃ 25.0 ± 0.4, on 120 mEq 26.9 ± 0.5 mEq/d [16]

Protection of Acid–Base Balance by pH Regulation of Acid Production

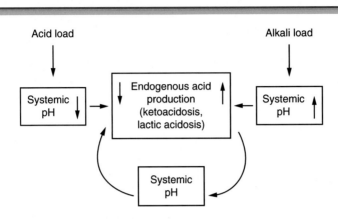

Fig. 7.6 Protection of acid–base balance by pH regulation of acid production. Addition of an acid load lowers organic acid production, thereby allowing the systemic pH to decrease, while addition of an alkali load increases organic acid production, increasing systemic pH [18]

($p=0.03$) [16]. When the bicarbonate was stopped, the plasma bicarbonate levels returned to baseline. In other words, the body reached a new set point for bicarbonate, dependent on the dose of bicarbonate given. In this study, blood hydrogen ion content decreased as plasma bicarbonate increased.

Although a change clearly occurs, how best to estimate the degree of change from dietary formulas is unclear. In a study in subjects with type 2 diabetes who were fed a diet very high in fruits and vegetables (which theoretically should be net base producing), NAE decreased significantly but did not decrease to the levels expected from the dietary formula estimates of NAE [17]. Possible explanations include higher-than-expected organic acid production and effects of diabetes on renal NAE.

Hood and Tannen suggested in 1998 [18] that systemic pH was protected by increasing or decreasing organic acid production in the direction that attenuates the change in systemic pH (Fig. 7.6). In overweight humans fasting or placed on ketogenic diets, addition of ammonium chloride (an acid) decreased urinary ketoacid excretion compared with the controls receiving sodium chloride, while those given sodium bicarbonate showed increased urinary ketoacid excretion. These studies suggest that alteration in organic acid production is one of the main methods the body uses to maintain systemic blood acid levels.

The "Trade-Off" Hypothesis

Robert Alpern in 1995 suggested that in order to maintain acid–base balance, the body accepts certain trade-offs (Fig. 7.7) [19]. In addition to the increase in ammonium excretion, the kidneys increase the reabsorption of citrate, leading to lower

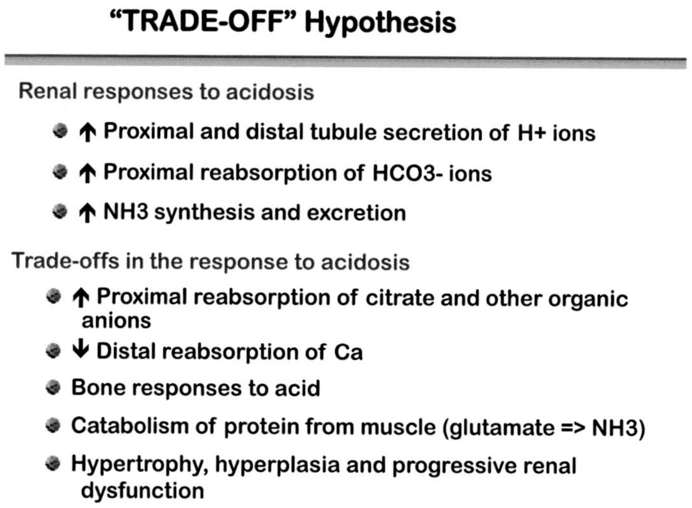

"TRADE-OFF" Hypothesis

Renal responses to acidosis

- ↑ Proximal and distal tubule secretion of H+ ions
- ↑ Proximal reabsorption of HCO3- ions
- ↑ NH3 synthesis and excretion

Trade-offs in the response to acidosis

- ↑ Proximal reabsorption of citrate and other organic anions
- ↓ Distal reabsorption of Ca
- Bone responses to acid
- Catabolism of protein from muscle (glutamate => NH3)
- Hypertrophy, hyperplasia and progressive renal dysfunction

Fig. 7.7 The "trade-off" hypothesis; to maintain systemic acid–base balance, the body must either neutralize or titrate the excess acids or bases, which over time could have pathophysiologic consequences [19]

urinary citrate levels; muscle protein breaks down to supply glutamate to the liver; and bones break down to supply alkali salts. In vitro studies demonstrate that at lower pH, muscle cells activate the ubiquitin-proteasome pathway, allowing the liver to increase glutamine production from glutamate, which in the renal proximal tubule is metabolized to alpha-ketoglutarate and ammonia [20]. Excretion of ammonia with a hydrogen ion (as ammonium, NH4+), is one of the main ways that the kidney can increase the excretion of metabolic acids. In bone, there is both a physico-chemical effect [21, 22] and a cellular effect, as osteoclasts (bone cells that break down bone) are activated to increase the release of base from hydroxyapatite [23].

Dietary Effects on Pathophysiologic Conditions

Many investigators have studied the effects of differing diet acid loads on mineral and endocrinologic systems in the body. Breslau et al. [24] fed young healthy subjects protein from vegetarian, vegetarian and egg, or animal protein and demonstrated that urinary calcium excretion increased as dietary acid load and NAE increased (Fig. 7.8). In this paper, the authors also noted that despite the increased urinary calcium excretion, serum parathyroid hormone (PTH) and 1,25 vitamin D levels decreased, with no change in intestinal calcium absorption. The authors suggested in this case, the higher serum calcium levels might be the cause of the depressed PTH and vitamin D. They further postulated that high acid diets leading to bone calcium loss might then be a risk factor for osteoporosis. Whether dietary

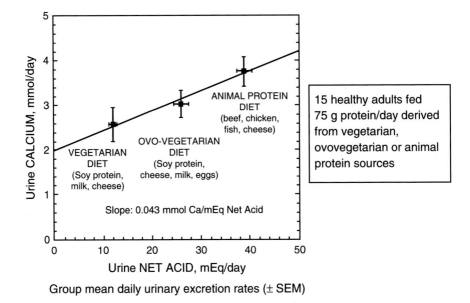

Group mean daily urinary excretion rates (± SEM)

Fig. 7.8 Fifteen young healthy subjects fed vegetarian, vegetarian and egg, or animal protein diets for 12 days. High protein diets were associated with higher uric acid excretion [24, 34]

acid intake is a factor in osteoporosis in otherwise healthy older subjects is both unclear and controversial [25, 26].

In addition, the high animal protein diets were associated with higher uric acid excretion. Reddy et al. [27] put healthy subjects on a severely carbohydrate restricted diet for 2 weeks and demonstrated decreases in urine pH and urinary citrate levels, and doubling of both urinary uric acid and urinary calcium excretion. These combinations of factors increase the risk for kidney stones. These effects are accentuated if the diet is also high in salt (NaCl), as high levels of NaCl also increase renal NAE, lower blood pH, and increase urinary calcium excretion [28]. In addition, subjects with diabetes when fed a high acid-producing diet have lower NAE and higher sulfate excretion than healthy volunteers fed the same diet, leading to a lower urinary pH [29].

Would eating a low acid diet or supplementing the diet with exogenous alkali therapy then help prevent these pathophysiologic consequences? For some of these problems, the answer is yes. In subjects with kidney stones that form at low urine pH (e.g., calcium oxalate and uric acid stones), lowering dietary salt intake, increasing calcium intake, lowering protein intake, and supplementing the diet with citrate if urinary citrate levels are low are standard therapies.

Low acid diets or supplementing the diet with exogenous alkali might also alter nitrogen loss and muscle mass in older subjects potentially at risk for falls [30]. One recent study suggested that alkali therapy could improve muscle function, as well as muscle mass in older men and women [31].

Recent studies by Wesson et al. [32, 33] also suggest that in subjects with mild renal insufficiency, supplementing the diet with sodium bicarbonate (NaHCO$_3$)

therapy permits the kidney to neutralize tissue acid loads, allowing the kidney to excrete a lower *net* acid load. Over time, this correlates with a slower decline in glomerular filtration rate in the group given $NaHCO_3$ compared with subjects given an equal amount of NaCl.

Question

Returning to the clinical vignette, the question was, should you agree that that patient can try the Atkins diet for weight loss?
    Which one of these BEST explains your response?

A. Yes, the Atkins diet has been shown to help subjects lose weight.
B. No, the Atkins diet is not a good diet for subjects with high blood sugar.
C. Yes, but you should tell her to increase her salt and water intake to help keep herself hydrated.
D. No, the Atkins diet can promote increased acid production and increase her risk for kidney stones.
E. No, the Atkins diet is contraindicated in subjects with high blood lipid levels.

    Answer: D

Explanation

The Atkins diet and its variants are low or very low carbohydrate diets, typically containing 20–50 "net carbs" (i.e., carbohydrate content minus fiber content) a day. Such diets often lower triglyceride levels dramatically, as well as lowering total and LDL cholesterol. These diets also improve fasting blood sugars and HgA1c. Therefore, answers B and E are incorrect. Increased water intake is recommended on a low carbohydrate diet, as well as for anyone at risk for developing kidney stones. Kidney stone incidence is increasing in women and is higher in areas with higher ambient temperature such as Florida. However, increasing salt intake would increase urinary calcium excretion, so C is incorrect. Although low carbohydrate diets often help people lose weight, this patient is diabetic and therefore at increased risk for kidney stones on a high protein diet, so D is a better answer than A.

References

1. Madias NE, Adrogué HJ, Horowitz GL, Cohen JJ, Schwartz WB. A redefinition of normal acid–base equilibrium in man: carbon dioxide tension as a key determinant of normal plasma bicarbonate concentration. Kidney Int. 1979;16(5):612–8.
2. Kurtz I, Maher T, Hulter HN, Schambelan M, Sebastian A. Effect of diet on plasma acid–base composition in normal humans. Kidney Int. 1983;24:670–80.

3. Frassetto LA, Morris Jr RC, Sebastian A. Dietary sodium chloride intake independently predicts the degree of hyperchloremic metabolic acidosis in healthy humans consuming a net acid-producing diet. Am J Physiol Renal Physiol. 2007;293:F521–5.

4. Frassetto LA, Morris Jr RC, Sebastian A. Effect of age on blood acid–base composition in adult humans: role of age-related renal functional decline. Am J Physiol. 1996;271(6 Pt 2):F1114–22.

5. Folin O. Laws governing the chemical composition of urine. Am J Physiol. 1905;13:66–115.

6. Sherman HC, Gettler AO. The balance of acid-forming and base-forming elements in foods, and its relation to ammonia metabolism. J Biol Chem. 1912;11:323–38.

7. Blatherwick NR. The specific role of foods in relation to the composition of the urine. Arch Int Med. 1914;14:409–50.

8. Relman AS, Lennon EJ, Lemann Jr J. Endogenous production of fixed acid and the measurement of the net balance of acid in normal subjects. J Clin Invest. 1961;40:1621–30.

9. Lennon EJ, Lemann Jr J, Relman AS. The effects of phosphoproteins on acid balance in normal subjects. J Clin Invest. 1962;41:637–45.

10. Lemann Jr J, Relman AS. The relation of sulfur metabolism to acid–base balance and electrolyte excretion: the effects of DL-methionine in normal man. J Clin Invest. 1959;38:2215–23.

11. Lennon EJ, Lemann Jr J. Influence of diet composition on endogenous fixed acid production. Am J Clin Nutr. 1968;21(5):451–6.

12. Lennon EJ, Lemann Jr J, Litzow JR. The effects of diet and stool composition on the net external acid balance of normal subjects. J Clin Invest. 1966;45(10):1601–7.

13. Remer T, Manz F. Estimation of the renal net acid excretion by adults consuming diets containing variable amounts of protein. Am J Clin Nutr. 1994;59:1356–61.

14. Frassetto LA, Todd KM, Morris Jr RC, Sebastian A. Estimation of net endogenous noncarbonic acid production in humans from diet potassium and protein contents. Am J Clin Nutr. 1998;68:576–83.

15. Sebastian A, Frassetto LA, Sellmeyer DE, Merriam RL, Morris Jr RC. Estimation of the net acid load of the diet of ancestral preagricultural Homo sapiens and their hominid ancestors. Am J Clin Nutr. 2002;76:1308–16.

16. Sebastian A, Harris ST, Ottaway JH, Todd KM, Morris Jr RC. Improved mineral balance and skeletal metabolism in postmenopausal women treated with potassium bicarbonate. N Engl J Med. 1994;330:1776–81.

17. Frassetto LA, Shi L, Schloetter M, Sebastian A, Remer T. Established dietary estimates of net acid production do not predict measured net acid excretion in patients with Type 2 diabetes on Paleolithic-Hunter-Gatherer-type diets. Eur J Clin Nutr. 2013;67(9):899–903.

18. Hood VL, Tannen RL. Protection of acid–base balance by pH regulation of acid production. N Engl J Med. 1998;339:819–26.

19. Alpern RJ. Trade-offs in the adaptation to acidosis. Kidney Int. 1995;47:1205–15.

20. May RC, Kelly RA, Mitch WE. Metabolic acidosis stimulates protein degradation in rat muscle by a glucocorticoid-dependent mechanism. J Clin Invest. 1986;77:614–21.

21. Bushinsky DA, Smith SB, Gavrilov KL, et al. Chronic acidosis-induced alteration in bone bicarbonate and phosphate. Am J Physiol Renal Physiol. 2003;285:F532–9.

22. Frick KK, Krieger NS, Nehrke K, et al. Metabolic acidosis increases intracellular calcium in bone cells through activation of the proton receptor OGR1. J Bone Miner Res. 2009;24:305–13.

23. Arnett TR, Dempster DW. Effect of pH on bone resorption by rat osteoclasts in vitro. Endocrinology. 1986;119:119–24.

24. Breslau NA, Brinkley L, Hill KD, Pak CY. Relationship of animal protein-rich diet to kidney stone formation and calcium metabolism. J Clin Endocrinol Metab. 1988;66(1):140–6.

25. Bonjour JP. Nutritional disturbance in acid–base balance and osteoporosis: a hypothesis that disregards the essential homeostatic role of the kidney. Br J Nutr. 2013;4:1–10.

26. Frassetto LA, Sebastian A. Commentary to accompany the paper entitled 'Nutritional disturbance in acid–base balance and osteoporosis: a hypothesis that disregards the essential homeostatic role of the kidney', by Jean-Philippe Bonjour. Br J Nutr. 2013;17:1–3.

27. Reddy ST, Wang CY, Sakhaee K, Brinkley L, Pak CY. Effect of low-carbohydrate high-protein diets on acid–base balance, stone-forming propensity, and calcium metabolism. Am J Kidney Dis. 2002;40(2):265–74.
28. Frings-Meuthen P, Baecker N, Heer M. Low-grade metabolic acidosis may be the cause of sodium chloride-induced exaggerated bone resorption. J Bone Miner Res. 2008;23(4):517–24.
29. Maalouf NM, Cameron MA, Moe OW, Sakhaee K. Metabolic basis for low urine pH in type 2 diabetes. Clin J Am Soc Nephrol. 2010;5:1277–81.
30. Mithal A, Bonjour JP, Boonen S, Burckhardt P, Degens H, El Hajj Fuleihan G, Josse R, Lips P, Morales Torres J, Rizzoli R, Yoshimura N, Wahl DA, Cooper C, Dawson-Hughes B, IOF CSA Nutrition Working Group. Impact of nutrition on muscle mass, strength, and performance in older adults. Osteoporos Int. 2013;24(5):1555–66.
31. Dawson-Hughes B, Castaneda-Sceppa C, Harris SS, Palermo NJ, Cloutier G, Ceglia L, Dallal GE. Impact of supplementation with bicarbonate on lower-extremity muscle performance in older men and women. Osteoporos Int. 2010;21(7):1171–9.
32. Wesson DE, Simoni J. Acid retention during kidney failure induces endothelin and aldosterone production which lead to progressive GFR decline, a situation ameliorated by alkali diet. Kidney Int. 2010;78(11):1128–35.
33. Wesson DE, Simoni J, Broglio K, Sheather S. Acid retention accompanies reduced GFR in humans and increases plasma levels of endothelin and aldosterone. Am J Physiol Renal Physiol. 2011;300(4):F830–7.
34. Lemann Jr J. Relationship between urinary calcium and net acid excretion as determined by dietary protein and potassium: a review. Nephron. 1999;81 Suppl 1:18–25.

Chapter 8
The Physiology of the Metabolic Acidosis of Chronic Kidney Disease (CKD)

Nimrit Goraya and Donald E. Wesson

Introduction

Metabolic acidosis is among the common complications of chronic kidney disease (CKD) and its prevalence increases with declining glomerular filtration rate (GFR) [1]. Because CKD is increasing in incidence and prevalence [2], clinicians increasingly face this metabolic disorder as a management challenge. Studies detailed elsewhere in this book support that its correction reduces its untoward complications. Management of metabolic acidosis is based in large part on understanding its physiology. Consequently, the full spectrum of health care providers, including those providing primary care, benefit by having a basic physiologic understanding of this physiology. This chapter gives a general overview of our understanding of the physiology of metabolic acidosis due to CKD.

Maintenance of Normal Acid–Base Homeostasis

Acidosis is a *process* in which body fluids experience a net gain of acid (H^+) or a loss of base (usually HCO_3), each leading to an increase in body fluid free H^+ concentration ($[H^+]$). When this process is caused by a decrease in the metabolic (HCO_3) component of the acid–base equilibrium ($[H^+] = PCO_2/[HCO_3] \times constant$), it is

N. Goraya, M.D.
Baylor Scott and White Health, Texas A&M Health Sciences Center College of Medicine,
2401 South 31st Street, Temple, TX 76508, USA
e-mail: ngoraya@sw.org

D.E. Wesson, M.D., M.B.A. (✉)
Baylor Scott and White Health, Department of Internal Medicine, Texas A&M Health
Sciences Center College of Medicine, 2401 South 31st Street, Temple, TX 76508, USA
e-mail: dwesson@sw.org

© Springer Science+Business Media New York 2016
D.E. Wesson (ed.), *Metabolic Acidosis*, DOI 10.1007/978-1-4939-3463-8_8

called metabolic acidosis. Many dietary components when metabolized and some metabolic processes impart acid challenges to normal acid–base status. This acid is initially buffered to minimize the change in body fluid pH (pH measures the concentration of free $H^+ = [H^+]$) that would otherwise occur. Nevertheless, the accumulated acid must eventually be excreted from the body to restore normal acid–base balance. In addition, other body processes might lead to a loss of HCO_3, and this lost HCO_3 must be regenerated to maintain normal body HCO_3 stores and thereby the integrity of this important buffer system. The serum profile characteristic of metabolic acidosis as a single (i.e., not part of a mixed acid–base disorder) is a reduced $[HCO_3]$ and reduced PCO_2, the latter being the physiologic response to the metabolic acidosis.

Acid–base balance is collaboratively maintained by the kidneys, lungs, and liver. Carbon dioxide (CO_2) gas, an end product of carbohydrate and fat metabolism, forms carbonic acid (H_2CO_3) in aqueous solution that dissociates to yield acid (H^+). This "volatile" H^+ is eliminated by the lungs. Amino acids of ingested dietary proteins are metabolized by the liver to yield H^+, base, or neither, depending upon the particular amino acid ingested. Diets typical of industrialized societies have a greater proportion of amino acids that when metabolized yield "fixed" H^+ and so, on balance, are H^+-producing [3]. This net endogenous acid production (NEAP), which averages ~1 meq/kg bw/day, must be balanced by urine net acid excretion (NAE) done by the kidney, to avoid progressive metabolic acidosis.

The kidney plays the major role in excretion of "fixed" or "non-volatile" acid and plays the major role in regenerating new HCO_3 to replace that lost through acid titration or lost from the body. The other major kidney contribution to maintenance of normal acid–base status is recovery of HCO_3 that is filtered into the kidney tubules; HCO_3 loss in the urine would itself lead to metabolic acidosis as noted. Consequently, kidneys play a major role in the body's defense against fixed H^+ acid gain and base loss as part of maintaining normal acid–base status. Let's first discuss how the body, and particularly the kidney, helps avoid sustained metabolic acidosis in the context of these ongoing challenges to acid–base status.

Body Response to Addition of Non-Volatile or "Fixed" Acid

Respiratory Response

The equation describing acid–base equilibrium ($[H^+] = PCO_2/[HCO_3] \times constant$) mathematically shows that the body can minimize the increase in body fluid $[H^+]$ that would otherwise occur in response to a decrease in $[HCO_3]$ that occurs with addition of fixed acid by concomitantly decreasing PCO_2. The necessary qualitative and quantitative increase in ventilation by the lungs is the same for the metabolic acidosis of CKD as in non-CKD causes of metabolic acidosis despite the uremic milieu that might adversely affect this response [4].

Buffering

Body systems can ameliorate the effect of added fixed acid to increase body fluid [H^+] (which is equivalent to a decrease in body fluid pH) and decrease in body fluid [HCO_3] by employing the HCO_3/H_2CO_3 buffer system and/or by binding the added H^+ to non-HCO_3 buffers, most notably hemoglobin and albumin. When residual kidney function is sufficient and/or the fixed acid load does not overwhelm the kidney's ability to excrete it and regenerate new HCO_3 to replace that which was titrated by the added fixed acid, body fluid [HCO_3] is only temporarily reduced, [HCO_3] is returned to normal, and body HCO_3 stores remain normal. When metabolic acidosis is sustained because kidney fixed acid excretory capacity is compromised and/or the fixed acid load exceeds normal kidney capacity to excrete it, metabolic acidosis is characterized by low extracellular and intracellular [HCO_3] and therefore low total body HCO_3 stores. With chronic metabolic acidosis, bone HCO_3 stores are also reduced [5]. It follows that patients with chronic metabolic acidosis have reduced HCO_3-mediated buffering capacity. Because CKD patients are commonly anemic, these patients also have lower non-HCO_3 buffer capacity than control patients. Consequently, CKD patients with metabolic acidosis and anemia have reduced acid-buffering capacity and therefore depend proportionately more on H^+ excretion (and proportionately less on H^+ buffering) than patients without either CKD or metabolic acidosis to maintain baseline acid–base homeostasis. We will see that CKD patients with reduced GFR have reduced capacity to excrete a fixed acid load. The combination of reduced acid-excretory capacity and reduced buffer capacity positions CKD patients for chronic metabolic acidosis.

H^+ Excretion

Dietary H^+ challenges to acid–base status of experimental animals [6] and humans [7] prompt the kidney to increase urine NAE in an effort return acid–base status to baseline. Urine NAE is generally expressed as: urine ammonium (NH_4^+) + urine titratable acid (TA) excretion − urine HCO_3 excretion.

- Urinary ammoniogenesis—accounts for about two-thirds of UNAE under the baseline conditions of the high-acid diet ingested by most individuals living in industrialized societies. Glutamine is converted to two molecules of urine NH_4^+ and HCO_3, respectively. For every molecule of NH_4^+ excreted, one new molecule of HCO_3 is generated.
- TA—refers to the process whereby the kidney excretes H^+ with non-NH_4^+ urinary buffers. To quantitate this, urine is titrated with alkali to raise the acid urine pH to that of blood. The amount of alkali necessary to increase urine pH to that of blood is TA. About one-third of UNAE is attributed to TA, with phosphate being the predominant buffer.

- HCO_3 excretion—under normal physiology, about 4500 mEq of HCO_3^- is filtered per day, with 80 % reabsorption in proximal tubule and net excretion in
  urine typically near zero when eating the high-acid-producing diet typical of
  industrialized societies.

Although not commonly included in most analyses, excretion of organic acids
like citrate also contributes to overall urine NAE [8]. Metabolism of citrate to CO_2
and H_2O consumes 2 or 3 H^+ (depending on whether it is citrate^{2-} or citrate^{3-} that is
metabolized) and so its metabolism yields two or three HCO_3 [9]. Consequently, its
urine loss is equivalent to HCO_3 loss. As mentioned, diets in industrialized societies
are typically acid-producing [3] and such diets are associated with low levels of
urine citrate excretion [10]. In addition, metabolic acidosis reduces this basal low
level further to near zero [8]. For this reason, it is commonly not included in the
calculation of urine NAE. This reduced urine citrate excretion in response to acid-
producing diets and to metabolic acidosis is mediated by augmented proximal
tubule citrate reabsorption [11].

The increment in urine NAE in response to dietary H^+ is mediated quantitatively
more by an increase in urine NH_4^+ excretion and less so by changes in excretion of
the remaining components of urine NAE, i.e., TA (increases in which will increase
urine NAE) and HCO_3 (decreases in which will increase urine NAE) [8]. Cumulative
urine NAE excretion in response to a chronic dietary acid challenge is less than the
quantity of administered acid in human subjects [5], suggesting net retention of
administered acid. Net acid retention measured by microdialysis occurs in experimental animals given a chronic dietary acid challenge and does not resolve until the
dietary acid challenge is discontinued [12]. These experimental animals maintained
plasma acid–base parameters not different from controls not given dietary acid [12].
Even substantial and sustained dietary acid challenges given to human subjects with
normal GFR cause only modest changes in plasma acid–base parameters from baseline, and these changes typically occur within the normal range of these plasma
measures of acid–base status [13]. Consequently, human subjects eating the typically high-acid-producing diets of industrialized societies [3] might have acid retention and suffer its adverse consequences even when plasma acid–base parameters
are within "normal," i.e., without plasma acid-base parameters that are consistent
with metabolic acidosis. This hypothesis is supported by studies showing that oral
alkali improved mineral balance and bone metabolism in elderly women with osteoporosis but without metabolic acidosis [14].

H^+ Excretion in the Setting of Normal GFR

Studies in experimental animals with normal baseline GFR show that measurable
increases in proximal tubule acidification occur in response to supra-physiologic
acid challenges, often induced with intravenous infusion and/or gastric gavage of
mineral acid [6]. Animals, however, do not typically face acid challenges of such

magnitude nor do humans typically face the equivalent magnitude of such challenges. By contrast, more modest acid challenges induced by dietary means, that are more typical of those that animals or humans might face, induce measurable changes in net distal nephron acidification without measurable changes in net proximal nephron acidification [15–18]. These studies support the relative greater importance of enhanced distal nephron compared to proximal nephron acidification in mediating kidney fixed H^+ excretion in the setting of the magnitude of acid challenges that animals, and importantly humans, are more likely to face. Acid challenges increase proximal tubule NH_4^+ production and delivery to more distal nephron segments [6] to constitute the necessary increment in urine NH_4^+ excretion and thereby increase in urine NAE described earlier. This increase in net distal nephron acidification is mediated by increased H^+ secretion [15–18] and decreased HCO_3 secretion [15, 17, 18]. The H^+-secreting distal nephron transporters whose activity is increased in response to a dietary H^+ load include the H^+-ATPase and the Na^+/H^+ exchanger but these in vivo studies detected no increase in activity of the H^+, K^+-ATPase [17, 18] in this setting. These changes in distal nephron acidification are induced in part by increased kidney action and levels of angiotensin II [19], aldosterone [18], and endothelin [16–18]. The increase in urine NAE in response to an acid challenge in patients with normal GFR is mediated by an increase in urine excretion of both NH_4^+ and TA but by a proportionately greater increase in NH_4^+ excretion [5].

H^+ Excretion in the Setting of Reduced GFR

The prevalence of metabolic acidosis increases in CKD as GFR declines [1, 20]. The Nephro Test Study Group showed as GFR decreased from 60 to 90 to <20 mL/min/1.73 m^2, prevalence of metabolic acidosis increased from 2 to 39 % [20]. In a cohort of more than 570,000 US veterans with non-dialysis-dependent CKD stages 1–5, there was a linear increase in the prevalence of patients with serum $[HCO_3]$ <22 mEq/L in patients with more advanced stages of CKD [21]. Importantly, the MESA study showed that lower serum $[HCO_3]$ was associated with more rapid kidney function decline, independent of GFR and albuminuria, in subjects with GFR > 60 mL/min/1.73 m^2 [22]. These latter data suggest that metabolic acidosis is a predictor of more rapid nephropathy progression, a topic covered in greater detail elsewhere in this book.

The mechanism mediating reduced GFR of most CKD patients is gradual destruction of functioning nephrons. This gradual rather than abrupt GFR loss allows time for remaining intact nephrons to increase function, including increased per nephron acid excretion, in an effort to maintain normal overall acid–base homeostasis. To maintain stable H^+ content of body fluids, patients with chronically reduced GFR who continue to eat diets of the same H^+ content as when their GFR was normal must either (1) mount the same overall urine NAE as when their GFR was normal as some CKD patients appear able to do [23, 24]; or (2) use an internal buffer source such as bone as other CKD patients apparently do [5]. Despite the acid-producing diets of industrialized societies [3], most such CKD patients appear to avoid progressive metabolic acidosis if they maintain GFR above 20–25 % of normal [25, 26], whichever mechanism (or both) they employ. Nevertheless, diets of very high H^+ content might induce metabolic acidosis at reduced GFRs above this level [27], particularly in elderly persons whose serum creatinine might reflect much lower GFR compared to younger individuals with the same serum creatinine [28].

When functioning nephron mass decreases progressively below 20–25 % of normal, overall urine NAE progressively decreases [29–31]. Among the components of urine NAE (NH_4^+, TA, HCO_3), reduced urine NH_4^+ excretion is the predominant mediator of reduced urine NAE in CKD with reduced GFR [23, 29–33]. Reduced ammonia (NH_3) production is due to the reduction in nephron mass [6], particularly the proximal tubule where most NH_3 is produced [33]. Nevertheless, reduced urine TA excretion also contributes at very low GFR levels [24]. Reduced urine NAE, and not increased NEAP, is the predominant mechanism for metabolic acidosis due to reduced GFR [30]. Compared to patients with normal GFR, those with reduced GFR have compromised ability increase urine NH_4^+ in response to an acid challenge [31]. These data support reduced urine NH_4^+ production and excretion as the single most important contributor to metabolic acidosis due to reduced GFR.

Because many patients do not reduce dietary acid intake as GFR decreases and therefore as urine NAE falls, urine NAE might decrease below NEAP and lead to progressive H^+ retention, with or without serum acid–base parameters reflective of metabolic acidosis. Recent human studies showed that urine NH_4^+ excretion, as well as overall urine NAE, decreased as GFR declined but NEAP did not decrease with declining GFR [34]. Interestingly, most patients in whom urine NAE decreased below NEAP did not experience a decrease in serum [HCO_3]. These recent data support that CKD patients develop progressive net acid retention as GFR declines, even when plasma acid–base parameters do not reflect metabolic acidosis [34]. Studies showing that patients given fixed H^+ excrete less H^+ than the administered H^+ load also suggest net H^+ retention [5]. Animal studies support that this net H^+ retention in response to dietary H^+ is greater in animals with reduced compared to normal GFR [35, 36]. This association of acid retention with reduced GFR, even without plasma acid–base parameters reflective of metabolic acidosis, is strengthened by animal studies using direct measurement of acid retention using microdialysis [35–37] and supported by other human studies assessing the presence of acid retention using indirect techniques [38]. This apparent acid retention occurs even though per unit of GFR, and presumably nephron H^+ excretion, appears to be enhanced [23, 24].

Urine NAE is largely a function of the distal nephron [39] and so increased per nephron urine NAE in patients with reduced GFR involves enhanced distal nephron function. Stimulated distal nephron acidification generally involves (1) increased luminal NH_4^+ secretion [40] to allow for increased urine NAE as previously described; (2) increased net HCO_3 reabsorption [41] consistent with increased H^+ secretion that promotes NH_4^+ secretion [40], titrates non-HCO_3 buffers, and reclaims remaining HCO_3, all of which promotes urine NAE; and (3) reduced HCO_3 delivery to the terminal distal nephron [6] which also favors NH_4^+ secretion [40] and permits secreted H^+ bring about acid excretion rather than HCO_3 reclamation. Studies in experimental CKD models show that each of these criteria is met. Such animals with CKD in vivo have increased NH_4^+ secretion into the lumen of distal nephron epithelia [42], have increased net HCO_3 reabsorption [6, 43–47], and have reduced HCO_3 delivery to the terminal distal nephron due in large measure to increased proximal tubule acidification [45]. Increased distal nephron acidification in experimental CKD models is mediated in part by increased kidney activity of AII [43, 44, 47], aldosterone [47], and endothelin [45, 47].

Interestingly, increased per nephron acidification is observed in animals with GFR low enough to be associated with metabolic acidosis [6, 42–45] as well as in those with less severely reduced GFR without metabolic acidosis [47]. Net acid retention associated with reduced GFR induces increased acidification in animals with reduced GFR without metabolic acidosis [47]. Augmented nephron acidification in the setting of reduced GFR is mediated in part by acid retention-induced increased levels of AII [47], aldosterone [36, 47], and endothelin [36, 47].

Excretion of NH_4^+ requires H^+ secretion, particularly in the distal nephron, and overall H^+ secretion is limited by the reduction in functioning nephron mass that mediates reduced GFR in CKD. Overall H^+ secretion might also be limited by reduced integrity of remaining tubule epithelia and/or by level of hormonal mediators that enhance H^+ secretion. Inflammatory diseases, particularly that involve the kidney interstitium, can damage tubule H^+ transporters and thereby limit H^+ excretion needed for NH_4^+ excretion [48]. Consequently, patients with diseases that cause damage to the kidney interstitium might develop metabolic acidosis at higher residual GFR than those without such diseases [48]. On the other hand, patients with reductions in hormones that stimulate H^+ secretion, like aldosterone, might also develop metabolic acidosis at higher GFR levels than those with normal hormone levels and activity [49].

Conclusions

Patients with CKD and reduced GFR have reduced ability to excrete endogenously produced or exogenously administered acid. When the fixed, as opposed to the "volatile" acid, challenge exceeds the kidney's ability to excrete it, acid retention ensues and can be manifest by changes in serum acid–base parameters that clinicians recognize as metabolic acidosis. Some recent data support that patients with reduced GFR might have acid retention without serum acid–base parameters reflective of metabolic acidosis and continuing research will help confirm this possibility and if confirmed, determine its clinical meaning. Reduced urine NAE excretion is mediated predominantly by reduced NH_4^+ production and excretion.

References

1. Hsu CY, Chertow GM. Elevations of serum phosphorus and potassium due to mild to moderate chronic renal insufficiency. Nephrol Dial Transplant. 2002;17:1419–25.
2. US Renal Data System: USRDS 2012 Annual Data Report. Bethesda, MD: The National Institutes of Health, National Institute of Diabetes and Digestive and Kidney Diseases; 2012.
3. Remer T. Influence of nutrition on acid–base balance-metabolic aspects. Eur J Nutr. 2001;40:214–20.
4. Ypersele de Strihou C, Frans A. The pattern of respiratory compensation in chronic uraemic acidosis. The influence of dialysis. Nephron. 1970;7:37–50.
5. Lemann Jr J, Bushinsky DA, Hamm LL. Bone buffering of acid and base in humans. Am J Physiol. 2003;285:F811–32.
6. Buerkert J, Martin D, Trigg D. Segmental analysis of the renal tubule in buffer production and net acid formation. Am J Physiol. 1983;244(Renal Fluid Electrolyte Physiol. 13):F442–54.
7. Lemann Jr J, Lennon EJ, Goodman Jr AD, Relman AS. The net balance of acid in subjects given large loads of acid or alkali. J Clin Invest. 1965;44:507–17.
8. Curthoys NP, Moe OW. Proximal tubule function and response to acidosis. Clin J Am Soc Nephrol. 2013. doi:10.2215/CJN.10391012.
9. Moe OW, Preisig PA. Dual role of citrate in mammalian urine. Curr Opin Nephrol Hypertens. 2006;15:419–24.
10. Mandel EI, Taylor EN, Curhan GC. Dietary and lifestyle factors and medical conditions associated with urine citrate excretion. Clin J Am Soc Nephrol. 2013;8:901–8.
11. Pajor AM. Sequence and functional characterization of a renal sodium/dicarboxylate cotransporter. J Biol Chem. 1995;270:5779–85.
12. Wesson DE. Dietary acid increases blood and renal cortical acid content in rats. Am J Physiol. 1998;274(Renal Physiol. 43):F97–103.
13. Kurtz I, Maher T, Hulter HN, et al. Effect of diet on plasma acid–base composition in normal humans. Kidney Int. 1983;24:670–80.
14. Sebastian A, Harris ST, Ottaway JH, Todd KM, Morris Jr RC. Improved mineral balance and skeletal metabolism in postmenopausal women treated with potassium bicarbonate. New Engl J Med. 1994;330:1776–81.
15. Wesson DE. Reduced HCO₃ secretion mediates increased distal nephron acidification induced by dietary acid. Am J Physiol 1996;271(Renal Fluid and Electrolyte Physiol. 40):F670–8.
16. Wesson DE. Endogenous endothelins mediate increased distal tubule acidification induced by dietary acid in rats. J Clin Invest. 1997;99:2203–11.
17. Khanna A, Simoni J, Hacker C, Duran M-J, Wesson DE. Increased endothelin activity mediates augmented distal nephron acidification induced by dietary protein. J Am Soc Nephrol. 2004;15:2266–75.
18. Khanna A, Simoni J, Wesson DE. Endothelin-induced increased aldosterone activity mediates augmented distal nephron acidification as a result of dietary protein. J Am Soc Nephrol. 2005;16:1929–35.
19. Levine DZ, Iacovitti M, Buckman S, Harrison V. In vivo modulation of rat distal tubule net HCO₃⁻ flux by VIP, isoproterenol, angiotensin II, and ADH. Am J Physiol Renal Fluid Electrolyte Physiol. 1994;266:F878–83.
20. Moranne O, Froissart M, Rossert J, Gauci C, Boffa JJ, Haymann JP, M'rad MB, Jacquot C, Houillier P, Stengel B, Fouqueray B. Timing of onset of CKD-related metabolic complications. J Am Soc Nephrol. 2009;20:164–71.
21. Kovesdy CP, Lott EH, Lu JL, et al. Hyponatremia, hypernatremia, and mortality in patients with chronic kidney disease with and without congestive heart failure. Circulation. 2012;125:677–84.
22. Driver TH, Shlipak MG, Katz R, Goldenstein L, Sarnak MJ, Hoofnagle AN, Siscovick DS, Kestenbaum B. Low serum bicarbonate and kidney function decline: the multi-ethnic study of atherosclerosis. Am J Kidney Dis. 2014;64:534–41.

23. MacClean AJ, Hayslett JP. Adaptive change in ammonia excretion in renal insufficiency. Kidney Int. 1980;17:595–606.
24. Goodman AD, Lemann Jr J, Lennon EJ, Relman AS. Production, excretion, and net balance of fixed acid in patients with renal failure. J Clin Invest. 1980;17:595–606.
25. Widmer B, Gerhardt RE, Harrington JT, Cohen JJ. Serum electrolytes and acid base composition: the influence of graded degrees of chronic renal failure. Arch Intern Med. 1979;139:1099–102.
26. Hakim R, Lazarus JM. Biochemical parameters in chronic renal failure. Am J Kidney Dis. 1988;11:238–47.
27. Adeva MM, Souto G. Diet-induced metabolic acidosis. Clin Nutr. 2011;30:416–21.
28. Frassetto LA, Todd K, Morris Jr RC, Sebastian A. Estimation of net endogenous noncarbonic acid production in humans from diet potassium and protein contents. Am J Clin Nutr. 1998;68:576–83.
29. Simpson DP. Control of hydrogen ion homeostasis and renal acidosis. Medicine. 1971;50:503–41.
30. Schwartz WB, Hall PW, Hays RM, Relman AS. On the mechanism of acidosis in chronic renal disease. J Clin Invest. 1959;38:39–52.
31. Welbourne T, Weber M, Bank N. The effect of glutamine administration on urinary ammonium excretion in normal subjects and patients with renal disease. J Clin Invest. 1972;51:1852–60.
32. Tizianello A, DeFerrari G, Garibotto G, Gurreri G, Robaudo C. Renal metabolism of amino acids and ammonia in subjects with normal renal function and in patients with chronic renal insufficiency. J Clin Invest. 1980;65:1162–73.
33. Dass PD, Kurtz I. Renal ammonia and bicarbonate production in chronic renal failure. Miner Electrolyte Metab. 1990;16:308–14.
34. Vallet M, Metzger M, Haymann J-P, Flamant M, Gauci C, Theret E, Boffa J-J, Vrtovsnik F, Froissart M, Stengel B, Houillier P. Urinary ammonia and long-term outcomes in CKD. Kidney Int. doi:10.1038/ki.2015.52.
35. Wesson DE, Simoni J. Increased tissue acid mediates progressive GFR decline in animals with reduced nephron mass. Kidney Int. 2009;75:929–35.
36. Wesson DE, Simoni J. Acid retention during kidney failure induces endothelin and aldosterone production which lead to progressive GFR decline, a situation ameliorated by alkali diet. Kidney Int. 2010;78:1128–35.
37. Wesson DE, Jo C-H, Simoni J. Angiotensin II-mediated GFR decline in subtotal nephrectomy is due to acid retention associated with reduced GFR. Nephrol Dial Transp. 2014. doi:10.1093/ndt/gfu388.
38. Wesson DE, Simoni J, Broglio K, Sheather S. Acid retention accompanies reduced GFR in humans and increases plasma levels of endothelin and aldosterone. Am J Physiol. 2011;Renal Physiol. 300:F830–7.
39. Batlle DC, Kurtzman NA. Renal regulation of acid–base homeostasis: integrated response. In: Seldin DW, Giebisch G, editors. The kidney: physiology and pathophysiology. New York: Raven; 1985. p. 1547–848.
40. Knepper MA, Packer R, Good DW. Ammonium transport in the kidney. Physiol Rev. 1989;69:179–248.
41. Knepper MA, Good DW, Burg MB. Ammonia and bicarbonate transport by rat cortical collecting ducts perfused in vitro. Am J Physiol. 1985;249(Renal Fluid Electrolyte Physiol 18):F870–7.
42. Buerkert J, Martin D, Trigg D, Simon E. Effect of reduced renal mass on ammonium handling and net acid formation by the superficial and juxtaglomerullary nephron of the rat. Evidence for impaired reentrapment rather decreased production of ammonium on the acidosis of uremia. J Clin Invest. 1983;71:1661–75.
43. Levine DZ, Iaocovitti M, Buckman S, et al. Ang II-dependent HCO_3 reabsorption in surviving rat distal tubules: expression/activation of H^+-ATPase. Am J Physiol. 1997;272(Renal Physiol. 41):F799–808.

44. Levine DZ, Iaocovitti M, Luck B, et al. Surviving rat distal tubule bicarbonate reabsorption: effects of chronic AT$_1$ blockade. Am J Physiol. 2000;278(Renal Physiol. 47):F476–83.
45. Wesson DE. Endogenous endothelins mediate augmented acidification in remnant kidneys. J Am Soc Nephrol. 2001;12:1826–35.
46. Phisitkul S, Hacker C, Simoni J, et al. Dietary protein causes a decline in the glomerular filtration rate of the remnant kidney mediated by metabolic acidosis and endothelin receptors. Kidney Int. 2008;73:192–9.
47. Wesson DE, Jo C-H, Simoni J. Angiotensin II receptors mediate increased distal nephron acidification caused by acid retention. Kidney Int. 2012;82:1184–94.
48. Batlle DC. Segmental characterization of defects in collecting tubule acidification. Kidney Int. 1986;30:546–53.
49. Schambelan M, Sebastian A, Biglieri EG. Prevalence, pathogenesis, and functional significance of aldosterone deficiency in hyperkalemic patients with chronic renal insufficiency. Kidney Int. 1980;17:89–101.

Chapter 9
Metabolic Acidosis and Cardiovascular Disease

Jeffrey A. Kraut and Glenn T. Nagami

Case

A 68-year-old man with history of diabetes mellitus is admitted with fever and decreased mental status. On examination he is found to be obtunded with a blood pressure of 100/60 mmHg, T 101.2 °F, and rales detected on physical examination of the left chest. Laboratory studies show the following: WBC count 25,000 with shift to the left; Na^+, 133 mEq/l; K^+, 5.8 mEq/l; HCO_3^-, 8 mEq/l; BUN, 50 mg/dl; creatinine, 2.5 mg/dl; pH, 7.02, PCO_2, 32 mmHg.

This patient has hypobicarbonatemia, acidemia, and hypocapnia. For this patient's degree of metabolic acidosis, his expected PCO_2 is 18–22 mmHg. Because his measured PCO_2 is 32 mmHg, his respiratory response is less robust than anticipated, indicating the presence of respiratory acidosis in addition to his apparent metabolic acidosis.

The most appropriate therapy for this patient is:

A. Supportive measures only
B. Intravenous sodium bicarbonate
C. THAM
D. Dialysis

J.A. Kraut, M.D. (✉)
Division of Nephrology, VHAGLA Healthcare System,
11301 Wilshire Boulevard, Los Angeles, CA 90073, USA
e-mail: jkraut@ucla.edu

G.T. Nagami, M.D. (✉)
Medicine and Research Services, VA Greater Los Angeles Healthcare System,
11301 Wilshire Boulevard, Los Angeles, CA 90073, USA

Department of Medicine, David Geffen School of Medicine at UCLA,
11301 Wilshire Boulevard, Los Angeles, CA 90073, USA
e-mail: glenn.nagami@va.gov

© Springer Science+Business Media New York 2016
D.E. Wesson (ed.), *Metabolic Acidosis*, DOI 10.1007/978-1-4939-3463-8_9

E. THAM and dialysis
F. C, D, or E

We will discuss the suggested approach to this case after our detailed discussion at the end of this chapter.

Introduction

Metabolic acidosis can be acute (lasting minutes to a few days) or chronic (lasting weeks to years) in nature. The adverse effects of these two forms of metabolic acidosis are distinctly different as are the benefits and complications of treatment. For example, abnormalities in cardiovascular function, including hemodynamic parameters, are prominent with acute metabolic acidosis thereby contributing to a high mortality rate [1]. By contrast, although there is an increased risk of death with chronic metabolic acidosis [2], there is no evidence that cardiovascular function is significantly compromised. There is however a link between metabolic acidosis and the stimulation of factors that could lead to cardiovascular disease, such as hypertension [3] and chronic inflammation [4]. Possibly a more focused assessment will reveal a closer relationship between metabolic acidosis and development of cardiovascular disease, but such studies have yet to be published.

In this chapter, we detail the abnormalities in cardiovascular function noted with both acute and chronic metabolic acidosis, their potential pathogenesis, and the impact of therapy.

General Differences Between Acute and Chronic Metabolic Acidosis

The distinction between acute and chronic metabolic acidosis is imprecise. In some studies, acute metabolic acidosis is defined as an acid–base disturbance lasting minutes to a few days in duration. By contrast, chronic metabolic acidosis is considered to last 3 days or more in duration. However, others define chronic metabolic acidosis as an acid–base disturbance lasting weeks to years [1]. The latter definition likely has more relevance for clinical situations and so this definition will be utilized in the present discussion.

The acidemia with acute metabolic acidosis is generally more severe than with chronic metabolic acidosis. With the former, blood pH can be as low as 6.8 but is usually above 7.3 with chronic metabolic acidosis and is never below 7.2 [5]. The less severe degree of acidemia presumably reflects the activation of body's defense mechanisms through the neutralization of acid by body buffers and the excretion of acid by the kidney. It is well accepted that the latter process requires several days to reach its maximum.

However, body buffering, which begins almost immediately, can also require several days to reach an optimal state, reflecting in part the recruitment of bone buffers [6].

The disorders producing acute and chronic metabolic acidosis are also usually different. The most common causes of acute metabolic acidosis are organic acidoses such as ketoacidosis and lactic acidosis, administration of large quantities of Cl^--rich solutions, and diarrhea [1]. By contrast, the most common cause of chronic metabolic acidosis is chronic kidney disease (CKD) or various forms of renal tubular acidosis [5]. Less frequently, chronic diarrhea or loss of bicarbonate-rich fluid from various intestinal fistulae leads to chronic metabolic acidosis.

These two critical factors, the severity of the acidemia and the duration of exposure of tissues to an acidic milieu, might account for the different clinical abnormalities observed with acute and chronic metabolic acidosis. Particularly, severity of the acidemia appears to be important in the genesis of cardiac dysfunction [7, 8] as described below. Nevertheless, there is a dearth of studies examining the impact of mild chronic metabolic acidosis on cardiac function, so that a deleterious effect of chronic metabolic acidosis on cardiac function cannot be completely ruled out.

Cardiovascular Effects of Acute Metabolic Acidosis

The major cardiovascular abnormalities observed in patients with acute metabolic acidosis are shown in Table 9.1. They are inferred from studies performed using cultured cells, isolated tissues, tissues perfused in vitro, whole animals, and in some cases humans [7–9].

Infusion of lactic acid or administration of phenformin to dogs with normal cardiac function designed to produce severe lactic acidosis (systemic pH < 7.2) caused a reduction in cardiac contractility and cardiac output [7, 8, 10]. Moreover, infusion of hydrochloric acid in rats produced peripheral vasodilatation and hypotension [9]. Central venoconstriction causing an increase in central blood volume has also been described. Although general vasodilatation of arterial vessels has often been reported, constriction of myocardial blood vessels, renal vessels, and pulmonary vessels has been reported with an acidic systemic pH [8].

Table 9.1 Major cardiovascular abnormalities observed in patients with acute metabolic acidosis

Adverse effects	Comments
Decreased cardiac contractility and cardiac output	Studies primarily in animals indicated decreased cardiac contractility observed when pH falls below 7.1–7.2
Cardiac arrhythmias	Frequency unknown
Hypotension	Related to decreased contractility and peripheral vasodilatation
Stimulation of inflammatory response	Noted with exposure of <24 h; major inflammatory mediators stimulated

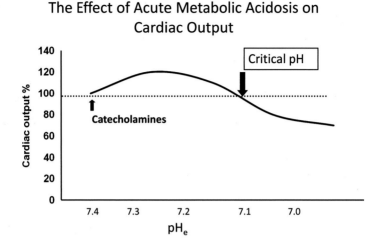

Fig. 9.1 The relationship between acute acidemia and cardiac function. As blood pH falls from 7.4 to 7.2, an increase in cardiac output can be observed. This is attributed to an influx of catecholamines, since it can be muted by administration of beta blockers. As systemic pH falls below 7.2, cardiac output falls by approximately 20 %. The fall in cardiac output might be greater in individuals with underlying cardiac disease or who are receiving beta blockers

The impairment of cardiovascular function with acute metabolic acidosis is clearly pH-dependent. As shown in Fig. 9.1, when systemic pH is reduced from 7.4 to 7.2 by the infusion of lactic acid, cardiac output actually rises [7, 10]. The rise in cardiac output is due to increased actions of catecholamines, since it was prevented by administration of beta blockers or prior removal of the adrenal glands. However, when systemic pH is reduced below 7.1–7.2, cardiac output falls, even in the presence of an intact sympathetic system. The response to endogenous or infused catecholamines is also muted thereby stemming the increment in cardiac output and peripheral resistance usually observed from the action of these hormones [8, 11]. On the other hand, vagal activity is stimulated particularly when systemic pH is reduced below <7.1 [8].

Metabolic acidosis also increases the risk for development of cardiac arrhythmias: their prevalence is higher both in the presence and absence of other factors that can provoke arrhythmias, such as changes in serum potassium or ionized calcium [12].

Oxygen delivery to tissues is also perturbed by metabolic acidosis. Experimentally induced metabolic acidosis leads to a rapid reduction in binding of oxygen to hemoglobin (Bohr effect) thereby improving tissue access to oxygen [13, 14]. Within 8 h, however, binding of oxygen to hemoglobin is enhanced somewhat by suppression of phosphofructokinase activity and resultant decreased net 2,3 diphosphoglycerate production (2,3 DPG). The final effect of acidosis on oxygen delivery depends on the sum of these counterbalancing forces, and therefore will depend on the duration of acidosis. The data support that a short duration of metabolic acidosis leads to decreased oxygen binding to hemoglobin, but hemoglobin oxygen binding appears to increase as the duration of metabolic acidosis increases.

Infusion of lactic acid in rats causes a decrease in cardiac cellular ATP levels [15]. This was presumed to be due to inhibition of a key enzyme involved in glycolysis, phosphofructose kinase (pH optimum of 7.2) [16, 17]. However, in this study the decreased cellular ATP levels were not associated with a significant fall in pH_i (7.13 vs 7.07 $p=NS$); observations suggesting that other factors might be involved in reducing ATP levels.

Metabolic acidosis alters the inflammatory response, an effect that could theoretically exacerbate or contribute to the development of cardiovascular dysfunction. Infusion of HCl to septic rats to produce severe non-anion gap (hyperchloremic acidosis) led to hypotension and an increased in the inflammatory molecules, IL-6, IL-10, and TNF [18]. Furthermore, exposure of cells to an acidic milieu increased expression of several pro-inflammatory cytokines within 24 h [4].

In summary, acute metabolic acidosis can reduce cardiac contractility and output, cause peripheral vasodilatation, and predisposes to arrhythmias, all of which favor the development of hypotension. These effects appear when blood pH is less than 7.2 in normal animals. Whether the same holds for humans has not been studied. Moreover, the aforementioned studies were performed in animals without underlying cardiovascular disease. Given the high prevalence of cardiovascular disease in the human population, it is likely that hemodynamic abnormalities would be observed more frequently in individuals with underlying cardiac disease. Even in the presence of more moderate acidosis, there will be increased outpouring of catecholamines which can increase peripheral resistance, cardiac contractility, and the threshold for appearance of arrhythmias. These observations suggest that in some cases, e.g., patients at high risk for arrhythmias, administration of base might be considered even with less severe acidemia.

Mechanisms of Cellular Dysfunction and Injury with Acute Metabolic Acidosis

Acute metabolic acidosis is associated with decreases in systemic, interstitial (pH_e), and intracellular pH (pH_i). Although cellular dysfunction with metabolic acidosis is attributed primarily to changes in pH_i, in vitro studies suggest that a reduction in pH_e can impair cellular function independent of any impact on pH_i [11]. Furthermore, administration of base to treat the acidosis might be successful in raising systemic pH while failing to raise intracellular or interstitial pH to the same extent, or paradoxically, even causing systemic and/or intracellular pH to fall transiently (particularly when base is given as sodium bicarbonate in patients with impaired tissue perfusion). Therefore, from a clinical perspective, there is some value in dividing the mechanisms underlying alterations in cellular function into those primarily related to a decrease in systemic and pH_e and those related to a decrease in pH_i, understanding that there can be significant overlap.

Effect of a Decrease in Extracellular pH (Table 9.2)

Table 9.2 Adverse effects of chronic metabolic acidosis

Adverse effect	Comments
Development or exacerbation of bone disease	Also leads to impaired growth in children
Degradation of muscle protein with muscle wasting	No evidence of effect on cardiac muscle
Reduced protein synthesis with tendency to hypoalbuminemia	Severe hypoalbuminemia could contribute to hypotension in patients particularly those on dialysis
Progression of chronic kidney disease	Related in part to increased endothelin and aldosterone levels that theoretically could affect hemodynamic function
Abnormalities of thyroid hormone synthesis	Alterations in levels could affect cardiac function
Development of hypertension	Suggestive relationship based on analysis of NHANES data
Increased production of aldosterone, endothelin, and catecholamines	Might contribute to genesis of cardiovascular disease

As discussed below, in addition to its impact on pH_i, a decrease in pH_e can theoretically impair cellular function and cause cell injury by attenuating cellular responsiveness to insulin and catecholamines. This effect of decreased pH_i and pH_e alters the opening of acid sensing ion channels (ASIC) in the brain and K channels in the heart and blood vessels, thereby activating proton-sensitive G-coupled receptors and activating transient receptor potential vanilloid 1 (TRPV1) channels in the heart and brain. Decreased pH_i and pH_e also alter activity of the CaSR receptor and increase the ionized component of intracellular and extracellular calcium concentration [19–21].

Acute metabolic acidosis is associated with impaired glucose tolerance and increased insulin resistance [19]; effects that can be reversed by correction of the acidosis. Although this might be related in part to a reduction in receptor number, binding of insulin to individual receptors is also impaired. The latter effect is related to the fall in interstitial pH, since exposure of isolated adipocytes to an extracellular $pH \leq 7.2$ reduced receptor binding of I^{125} insulin [22]. The magnitude of this decrease was correlated with the severity of the reduction in extracellular pH: receptor binding falling to 30–70 % of control values when extracellular pH was reduced to 6.7.

The blunted response of the cardiovascular system to catecholamines is due to a decrease in pH_i and pH_e. Prior exposure of neutrophil beta-adrenergic receptors to a low pH (7.1) leads to a striking reduction in isoproterenol-stimulated cAMP accumulation associated with decreased binding of catecholamine to its receptor [11].

The Ca^{2+}-sensing receptor is present in the heart and its sensitivity to Ca^{2+} and response to PTH were depressed by an acidic milieu. Activation of the calcium sensing receptor has been postulated to play a role in the magnitude of ischemia-reperfusion injury [23, 24].

Acid sensing ion channels (ASIC) ASIC1a, are pH-sensitive channels permeable to both calcium and sodium (half maximal activation at an external pH of 6.2–6.8) which are expressed at extremely high levels on dorsal root ganglion sensory neurons of the heart. They have been implicated in the transmission of ischemic pain. Since these channels are absent in cardiomyocytes, they presumably play no role in the cardiovascular response to acidosis [25]

Transient receptor potential vanilloid 1 (TRPV1) channels are Ca^{2+}-permeable channels expressed also in the heart that are activated by an external pH < 6.0. It has been postulated these channels might contribute to myocardial cell death and development of cardiac arrhythmias, particularly with severe metabolic acidosis [26].

Proton-sensing G-protein-coupled receptors such as OGR1 and G2A present in vascular tissue (half maximal activation at a pH_e of 7.17) cause release of Ca^{2+} from intracellular stores with subsequent IP_3 production. Their presence in vascular smooth muscle has led to speculation that their activation contributes to the arterial vasodilatation observed with metabolic acidosis, but this requires further examination [27].

Several potassium channels in the heart and vascular tissues are pH-sensitive [28]. Alterations of potassium flux thorough the channels might contribute to development of cardiac arrhythmias and hypotension with acute acidosis.

Finally, a reduction in systemic pH increases the concentration of ionized calcium by reducing its binding to albumin. The increase in Ca^{2+} has been postulated to counteract the depressive effect of a reduced pH on cardiac contractility.

Intracellular pH

A reduction in pH_i of the heart is postulated to play a dominant role in myocardial dysfunction. Decreased binding of Ca^{2+} to troponin and impaired enzyme activity reducing ATP production are major factors [29]. Activation of the Na^+-H^+ exchanger, NHE1 by acidosis might also contribute to cardiac dysfunction and development of arrhythmias, particularly with acute lactic acidosis [30]. Activation of NHE1 increases intracellular sodium and secondarily intracellular calcium leading to marked elevation of the concentration of both cations in myocardial cells [30]. Inhibition of NHE1 attenuates the increase in sodium and calcium and lessens the impact of acute lactic acidosis on cardiovascular function. Several studies have also demonstrated that administration of a selective inhibitor to animals with various models of lactic acidosis strikingly reduces mortality presumably related to improvement in cardiovascular function [31].

Response of the Heart to Administration of Base

Theoretically, administration of base would be expected to improve disturbed cardiovascular function through amelioration of the accompanying acidemia. However, administration of sodium bicarbonate depresses cardiovascular function in animal studies [32]. Moreover, although administration of base did not depress cardiac function in humans, its administration did not increase cardiac output more than an equivalent quantity of normal saline, despite significant increase in systemic pH induced by the administered base [33, 34]. The failure of bicarbonate to improve cardiac function despite an improvement of systemic pH has been attributed to two possible factors: (1) generation of carbon dioxide during the buffering process with rapid entry of carbon dioxide into myocardial cells and a decrease in pH_i [1]; and/or (2) a reduction in ionized calcium because of increased binding to albumin [33].

Based on these findings, it might be expected that administration of a base that did not generate significant quantities of carbon dioxide, and stabilization of ionized calcium by administration of calcium might allow expression of positive effects of correction of the acidosis. The latter possibility has been investigated with carbicarb, a 1:1 mixture of sodium bicarbonate and disodium carbonate [35]. In vitro studies involving addition of carbicarb to acidified blood led to a reduction in carbon dioxide [36]. Moreover, administration of carbicarb to dogs with metabolic acidosis improved cardiac function and pH_i [37]. Studies in humans were less impressive with only a subset of individuals having a positive response to carbicarb [38]. Further studies examining potential of carbicarb or other bases which consume carbon dioxide are under investigation.

At this juncture, the decision about what buffer to administer and what level of blood pH to target has not been resolved. It appears reasonable to target a blood pH of 7.2 as a goal since many of the adverse effects on the cardiovascular system are detected at this level as described above. If sodium bicarbonate is given, it should be administered as an isotonic solution at a slow rate. Since this can cause ionized Ca^{2+} to fall, administration of calcium is reasonable although this strategy has not been subject to rigorous examination. Utilization of THAM as an alternative needs to be examined more closely as does the use of dialysis. Furthermore, administration of NHE1 inhibitor as an adjunct to base therapy should be examined. Only with intense clinical investigation of different modalities of treatment will evidence-based guidelines be made available.

Chronic Metabolic Acidosis

The major adverse effects of chronic metabolic acidosis are shown in Table 9.2. Noticeable by their absence are abnormalities in cardiovascular function. In contrast to acute metabolic acidosis, no direct impact of chronic metabolic acidosis on cardiovascular function has been documented. It is not clear how meticulously investigators have approached this issue and it is possible that a relationship could be found. However, the less severe degree of acidemia in patients with chronic acidosis could explain, at least in part, the absence of cardiovascular abnormalities. As noted, no change in cardiac contractility is noted as blood pH is reduced from 7.4 to 7.2, and in vitro studies have predominately examined both increases and decreases at extreme levels of pH to determine the effect of pH changes in cellular function. Thus, the failure to observe cardiovascular abnormalities is not surprising.

One potential link between metabolic acidosis and abnormalities in cardiovascular function is the increase production of beta 2 microglobulin in dialysis patients with acidosis [39]. In patients with excess beta 2 microglobulin, there is greater deposition of amyloid in tissues, including the heart.

Also, recent studies suggest that metabolic acidosis is a risk factor for development of hypertension [3]. Among non-obese adult women, higher plasma bicarbonate was modestly associated with lower odds of developing hypertension after adjusting for matching factors. Also, hypertension was positively correlated with an increased dietary acid load [40]. Thus, either metabolic acidosis or an increase in an acid load, conditions theoretically characterized by increased tissue acidity were associated with a risk of hypertension; data consistent with acidosis or acid retention being a contributory factor for development of hypertension. On the other hand, in a separate large study there was no association between acid load and the risk for hypertension [41]. Further studies will be required to resolve this controversy. It is intriguing to think that increased tissue acidity contributes to hypertension, and if so it could represent an indirect link to development of cardiovascular disease.

Many investigators consider inflammation as a factor in the development of ischemic cardiovascular disease. Exposure of individual epithelial cell or macrophages to reductions in pH elicits an increase in the production and release of pro-inflammatory cytokines [4, 42]. These effects could contribute to the development of atherosclerotic cardiovascular disease.

Finally, in addition to enhanced production of catecholamines, investigators have documented an increase production of endothelin-1 and aldosterone [43]. All three hormones could affect cardiac remodeling or injury by various mechanisms. More intense investigations of these and other potential factors that might promote the development of cardiovascular disease are warranted.

Further evidence that metabolic acidosis might contribute to cardiovascular disease can be inferred from the increase in mortality of individuals with metabolic acidosis serum bicarbonate <17 mEq/l [2]. Since cardiovascular disease is the most common cause of mortality in patients with CKD both prior to and after initiation of chronic dialysis, it is reasonable to infer that chronic acidosis might contribute to development of cardiovascular disease with an eventual increase in mortality. Figure 9.2 presents a hypothetical model demonstrating how chronic acidosis might lead to cardiovascular disease and eventual increase in mortality.

In summary, chronic metabolic acidosis does not appear to produce acute cardiac dysfunction. However, it could promote the development of cardiovascular disease through its stimulation of key hormones that affect the cardiovascular system, and the development of hypertension.

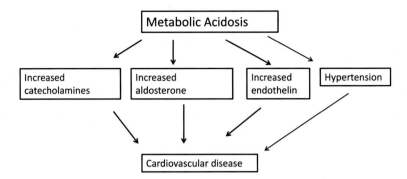

Fig. 9.2 Hypothetical relationship between chronic metabolic acidosis and cardiovascular disease. Chronic metabolic acidosis can be associated with stimulation of catecholamines, endothelin, and aldosterone. In addition to stimulation of these hormones, it can promote inflammation and the development of hypertension. The sum of these factors can lead to ischemic cardiovascular disease or cardiomyopathy

The Impact of Base on Cardiovascular Function with Chronic Metabolic Acidosis

Although metabolic acidosis itself appears not to be associated with cardiovascular dysfunction, some of its treatment strategies have been associated with adverse cardiovascular outcomes. A recent study found that in patients with CKD not on dialysis, a serum bicarbonate above 24 mEq/l due to diuretic administration or base therapy was associated with a marked increase in the prevalence of congestive heart failure [44, 45]

These findings suggest either that mild hypobicarbonatemia is protective against cardiovascular disease or, more likely, that an elevated plasma bicarbonate and pH is associated with cardiovascular dysfunction. Possibly, a more alkaline pH predisposes to calcifications which could contribute both to ischemic disease or cardiomyopathy [46]. Further studies to examine this issue are warranted, particularly since the elegant studies of Wesson's group [47–49] suggest that early base therapy is beneficial in slowing progression of CKD.

It appears very clear that administration of base is beneficial in patients with metabolic associated with CKD. Presently, recommendations are to administer base when serum [HCO_3^-] is less than 22 mEq/l [50, 51]. The precise goal is not clear although it seems reasonable to keep it less than 24 mEq/l. Base can be given as sodium bicarbonate, or sodium citrate. The former is associated with gas production in the stomach which can be bothersome for some patients. In both instances it is worthwhile estimating the base deficit by multiplying the difference between the prevailing serum [HCO_3^-] and the desired serum [HCO_3^-] × the space of distribution usually given as 50 % body weight (kg). The total base required can be given over several days. Once a serum [HCO_3^-] has been reached, the quantity of base should be reduced. In lieu of base, some investigators have demonstrated increasing the intake of fruits and vegetables is also effective [52]. There is, of course, the potential risk of hyperkalemia but this can be avoided by choosing patients who are at low risk for hyperkalemia and by careful observation of patients treated in this way. A reduction in animal-sourced protein intake will also reduce the net endogenous acid production and is an ancillary measure that is useful.

Returning to Our Case

Answers: F. C, D, or E

The treatment of acute metabolic acidosis is one of the most controversial issues in clinical medicine today [53]. Although it is well accepted that an acidic environment is associated with compromise of the cardiovascular system, the use of base to improve it has not been successful [1]. Sodium bicarbonate is associated with generation of carbon dioxide which exacerbates intracellular acidosis. Therefore, administration of bicarbonate in this patient with incipient carbon dioxide retention would theoretically be deleterious. Indeed, in a recent animal study, hyperventilation to prevent carbon dioxide retention was associated with improved cardiovascular response [54]. THAM can raise blood and intracellular pH without generating carbon dioxide. It is cleared by the kidney and therefore might have to be used cautiously in this case. Combining THAM administration and dialysis to remove THAM might be used. Dialysis alone which provides base in the form of sodium bicarbonate but can control volume and changes in osmolality might also be considered. Other measures such as administration of an NHE1 (Na^+-H^+ exchange) inhibitor are also under investigation [55]. In summary, the treatment of acute metabolic acidosis remains under investigation and individualized care will be necessary in the treatment of patients.

References

1. Kraut JA, Madias NE. Metabolic acidosis: pathophysiology, diagnosis and management. Nat Rev Nephrol. 2010;6(5):274–85.
2. Bommer J, Locatelli F, Satayathum S, et al. Association of predialysis serum bicarbonate levels with risk of mortality and hospitalization in the Dialysis Outcomes and Practice Patterns Study (DOPPS). Am J Kidney Dis. 2004;44(4):661–71.
3. Mandel EI, Forman JP, Curhan GC, Taylor EN. Plasma bicarbonate and odds of incident hypertension. Am J Hypertens. 2013;26(12):1405–12.
4. Raj S, Scott DR, Nguyen T, Sachs G, Kraut JA. Acid stress increases gene expression of proinflammatory cytokines in Madin-Darby canine kidney cells. Am J Physiol Renal Physiol. 2013;304(1):F41–8.
5. Kraut JA, Kurtz I. Metabolic acidosis of CKD: diagnosis, clinical characteristics, and treatment. Am J Kidney Dis. 2005;45(6):978–93.
6. Lemann J, Bushinsky DA, Hamm LL. Bone buffering of acid and base in humans. Am J Physiol. 2003;285(5):F811–32.

7. Wildenthal K, Mierzwiak DS, Myers RW, Mitchell JH. Effects of acute lactic acidosis on left ventricular performance. Am J Physiol. 1968;214:1352–9.
8. Mitchell JH, Wildenthal K, Johnson Jr RL. The effects of acid–base disturbances on cardiovascular and pulmonary function. Kidney Int. 1972;1(5):375–9.
9. Kellum JA, Song MC, Venkataraman R. Effects of hyperchloremic acidosis on arterial pressure and circulating inflammatory molecules in experimental sepsis. Chest. 2004;125(1):243–8.
10. Teplinsky K, Otoole M, Olman M, Walley KR, Wood LD. Effect of lactic acidosis on canine hemodynamics and left ventricular function. Am J Physiol. 1990;258(4):H1193–9.
11. Davies AO. Rapid desensitization and uncoupling of human beta adrenergic receptors in an in vitro model of lactic acidosis. J Clin Endocrinol Metab. 1984;59(3):398–405.
12. Orchard CH, Cingolani HE. Acidosis and arrhythmias in cardiac muscle. Cardiovasc Res. 1994;28(9):1312–9.
13. Bellingham AJ, Detter JC, Lenfant C. Regulatory mechanisms of hemoglobin oxygen affinity in acidosis and alkalosis. J Clin Invest. 1971;50(3):700–6.
14. Rolf LL, Garg LC. Effect of acetazolamide and carbonic anhydrase inhibition on erythrocyte 2,3-diphosphoglycerate content and metabolism. J Pharmacol Exp Ther. 1975;193(2):639–46.
15. Zahler R, Barrett E, Majumdar S, Greene R, Gore J. Lactic acidosis: effect of treatment on intracellular pH and energetics in living rat heart. Am J Physiol. 1992;262:H1572–8.
16. Halperin FA, Cheema-Dhadli S, Chen CB, Halperin MI. Alkali therapy extends the period of survival during hypoxia: studies in rats. Am J Physiol. 1996;271:R381–7.
17. Trivedi B, Danforth WH. Effect of pH on the kinetics of frog muscle phosphofructokinase. J Biol Chem. 1966;241:4110–4.
18. Kellum JA, Song MC, Almasri E. Hyperchloremic acidosis increases circulating inflammatory molecules in experimental sepsis. Chest. 2006;130(4):962–7.
19. Cuthbert C, Alberti KG. Acidemia and insulin resistance in the diabetic ketoacidotic rat. Metabolism. 1978;27:1903–16.
20. Kraut JA, Madias NE. Treatment of acute metabolic acidosis. Nephrol Nat Rev. 2012;8:589–601.
21. Quinn SJ, Bai M, Brown EM. pH sensing by the calcium-sensing receptor. J Biol Chem. 2004;279(36):37241–9.
22. Whittaker C, Cuthbert C, Hammond VA, Alberti KGMM. The effect of metabolic acidosis in vivo on insulin binding to isolated rat adipocytes. Metabolism. 1982;31:553–7.
23. Zhang WH, Fu SB, Lu FH, et al. Involvement of calcium-sensing receptor in ischemia/reperfusion-induced apoptosis in rat cardiomyocytes. Biochem Biophys Res Commun. 2006;347(4):872–81.
24. Guo J, Li HZ, Zhang WH, et al. Increased expression of calcium-sensing receptors induced by ox-LDL amplifies apoptosis of cardiomyocytes during simulated ischaemia-reperfusion. Clin Exp Pharmacol Physiol. 2010;37(3):e128–35.
25. Bethell HWL, Vandenberg JI, Smith GA, Grace AA. Changes in ventricular repolarization during acidosis and low-flow ischemia. Am J Physiol Heart Circ Physiol. 1998;44(2):H551–61.
26. Watanabe H, Murakami M, Ohba T, Ono K, Ito H. The pathological role of transient receptor potential channels in heart disease. Circ J. 2009;73(3):419–27.
27. Tomura H, Mogi C, Sato K, Okajima F. Proton-sensing and lysolipid-sensitive G-protein-coupled receptors: a novel type of multi-functional receptors. Cell Signal. 2005;17(12):1466–76.
28. Jiang C, Qu ZQ, Xu HX. Gating of inward rectifier K+ channels by proton-mediated interactions of intracellular protein domains. Trends Cardiovasc Med. 2002;12(1):5–13.
29. Garciarena CD, Youm JB, Swietach P, Vaughan-Jones RD. H(+)-activated Na(+) influx in the ventricular myocyte couples Ca(2+)-signalling to intracellular pH. J Mol Cell Cardiol. 2013;61:51–9.
30. Wu DM, Kraut JA. Potential role of NHE1 (sodium-hydrogen exchanger 1) in the cellular dysfunction of lactic acidosis: implications for treatment. Am J Kidney Dis. 2011;57(5):781–7.
31. Wu DM, Kraut JA, Abraham WM. Sabiporide improves cardiovascular function, decreases the inflammatory response, and reduces mortality in acute metabolic acidosis in pigs. PLoS One. 2013;8:e593932–8.
32. Graf H, Leach W, Arieff AI. Evidence for a detrimental effect of bicarbonate therapy in hypoxic lactic acidosis. Science. 1985;227:754–6.

33. Cooper DJ, Walley KR, Wiggs BR, Russell JA. Bicarbonate does not improve hemodynamics in critically ill patients who have lactic acidosis. Ann Intern Med. 1990;112(7):492–8.
34. Mathieu D, Neviere R, Billard V, Fleyfel M, Wattel F. Effects of bicarbonate therapy on hemodynamics and tissue oxygenation in patients with lactic acidosis: a prospective, controlled clinical study. Crit Care Med. 1991;19(11):1352–6.
35. Filley GF, Kindig NB. Carbicarb, an alkalinizing ion generating agent of possible clinical usefulness. Trans Am Clin Climatol Assoc. 1984;96:141–53.
36. Shapiro JI, Elkins N, Logan J, Ferstenberg LB, Repine JE. Effects of sodium-bicarbonate, disodium carbonate, and a sodium-bicarbonate carbonate mixture on the P-CO$_2$ of blood in a closed-system. J Lab Clin Med. 1995;126(1):65–9.
37. Shapiro JI, Whalen M, Chan L. Hemodynamic and hepatic pH responses to sodium-bicarbonate and carbicarb during systemic acidosis. Magn Reson Med. 1990;16(3):403–10.
38. Leung JM, Landow L, Franks M, et al. Safety and efficacy of intravenous Carbicarb in patients undergoing surgery: comparison with sodium bicarbonate in the treatment of metabolic acidosis. Crit Care Med. 1994;22(10):1540–9.
39. Sonikian M, Gogusev J, Zingraff J, et al. Potential effect of metabolic acidosis on beta 2-microglobulin generation: in vivo and in vitro studies. J Am Soc Nephrol. 1996;7(2):350–6.
40. Zhang L, Curhan GC, Forman JP. Diet-dependent net acid load and risk of incident hypertension in United States women. Hypertension. 2009;54(4):751–5.
41. Engberink MF, Bakker SJ, Brink EJ, et al. Dietary acid load and risk of hypertension: the Rotterdam study. Am J Clin Nutr. 2012;95(6):1438–44.
42. Kellum JA, Song MC, Li JY. Lactic and hydrochloric acids induce different patterns of inflammatory response in LPS-stimulated RAW 264.7 cells. Am J Physiol. 2004;286(4):R686–92.
43. Wesson DE, Simoni J. Increased tissue acid mediates a progressive decline in the glomerular filtration rate of animals with reduced nephron mass. Kidney Int. 2009;75(9):929–35.
44. Kraut JA, Madias NE. Association of serum bicarbonate with clinical outcomes in CKD: could an increase in serum bicarbonate be a double-edged sword? Am J Kidney Dis. 2013;62:647–9.
45. Dobre M, Yang W, Chen J. Association of serum bicarbonate with risk of renal and cardiovascular outcomes in chronic kidney disease. A report from the chronic renal insufficiency cohort (CRIC). Am J Kidney Dis. 2013;62:670–8.
46. Kraut JA, Madias NE. Consequences and therapy of the metabolic acidosis of chronic kidney disease. Pediatr Nephrol. 2011;26(1):19–28.
47. Goraya N, Simoni J, Hee-Jo C, Wesson DE. A comparison of treating metabolic acidosis in CKD stage 4 hypertensive kidney disease with fruits and vegetables or sodium bicarbonate. Clin J Am Soc Nephrol. 2013;8:3–11.
48. Goraya N, Wesson DE. Does correction of metabolic acidosis slow chronic kidney disease progression? Curr Opin Nephrol Hypertens. 2013;22(2):193–7.
49. Wesson DE, Simoni J. Acid retention during kidney failure induces endothelin and aldosterone production which lead to progressive GFR decline, a situation ameliorated by alkali diet. Kidney Int. 2010;78(11):1128–35.
50. National Kidney Foundation. K/DOQI clinical practice guidelines for nutrition in chronic renal failure. Am J Kidney Dis. 2000;35:S1–140.
51. KDIGO 2012 clinical practice guidelines for the evaluation and management of chronic kidney disease: Chapter 3. Kidney Int Suppl. 2013;3:73–90.
52. Goraya N, Simoni J, Jo CH, Wesson DE. A comparison of treating metabolic acidosis in CKD stage 4 hypertensive kidney disease with fruits and vegetables or sodium bicarbonate. Clin J Am Soc Nephrol. 2013;8:86–93.
53. Treatment of metabolic acidosis: controversies and challenges. NephSAP. 2015;14:1–6.
54. Kimmoun A, Ducrocq N, Sennoun N, Issa K, Strub C, Escamye JM. Efficient extra and intracellular alkalinization improves cardiovascular functions in severe lactic acidosis induced by hemorrhagic shock. Anaesthesiology. 2014;120:926–34.
55. Wu D, Kraut J. Role of NHE1 in the cellular dysfunction of acute metabolic acidosis. Am J Nephrol. 2014;40:36–42.

Chapter 10
Effects of Metabolic Acidosis on Skeletal Muscle

Afolarin Amodu and Matthew K. Abramowitz

Case: P.M. is a 56-year-old woman with stage 3 chronic kidney disease (CKD) due to longstanding type 2 diabetes mellitus and hypertension. She takes an angiotensin-receptor blocker and a beta-blocker, and her diabetes is managed with a dipeptidyl peptidase-4 inhibitor and oral agents including a thiazolidinedione. On exam, her blood pressure is 109/68 mmHg and she has no edema. Over the past year her kidney function has remained stable, with an estimated glomerular filtration rate of 30 mL/min/1.73 m². Her serum bicarbonate is 20 mEq/L and serum potassium is 4.5 mEq/L. She requires 24 s to complete 10 repetitions of a sit-to-stand-to-sit test, which is slower than the predicted time range for women of her age group. Would treatment with alkali therapy improve muscle strength and physical performance? How should this patient be managed?

(a) Begin oral sodium bicarbonate after confirming metabolic acidosis with a venous blood gas.
(b) Measure the serum bicarbonate again in 3 months; if unchanged, recommend increased intake of fruits and vegetables.

A. Amodu, M.D., M.P.H.
Division of Nephrology, Department of Medicine, Albert Einstein College of Medicine, 1300 Morris Park Avenue, Ullmann 615, Bronx, NY 10461, USA
e-mail: aaamodu@gmail.com

M.K. Abramowitz, M.D., M.S. (✉)
Division of Nephrology, Department of Medicine, Albert Einstein College of Medicine, 1300 Morris Park Avenue, Ullmann 615, Bronx, NY 10461, USA

Department of Epidemiology & Population Health, Albert Einstein College of Medicine, 1300 Morris Park Avenue, Ullmann 615, Bronx, NY 10461, USA
e-mail: matthew.abramowitz@einstein.yu.edu

© Springer Science+Business Media New York 2016
D.E. Wesson (ed.), *Metabolic Acidosis*, DOI 10.1007/978-1-4939-3463-8_10

(c) Measure the serum bicarbonate again in 3 months; if unchanged, prescribe oral sodium bicarbonate.
(d) Prescribe oral sodium bicarbonate 0.3 mEq/kg body weight/day in two divided doses.
(e) Prescribe oral sodium bicarbonate 1 mEq/kg body weight/day in two divided doses.

Introduction

Metabolic acidosis is highly prevalent in persons with advanced CKD. This is mainly due to reduced renal mass leading to impaired ammoniagenesis and inability to excrete the daily acid load. As bone is the most important buffer of a chronic acid load, bone resorption in response to chronic acidosis is not surprising. Less well recognized by clinicians are changes in muscle metabolism in response to chronic metabolic acidosis.

The catabolic effects of chronic acidosis can be subtle and thus easily overlooked by clinicians. This has important implications, as skeletal muscle wasting is associated with increased morbidity and mortality [1]. Furthermore, the effects of acidosis are not only relevant to the population with kidney disease. A low-level acidosis, related to older age and high net endogenous acid production due to the Western diet, may be of importance in individuals without CKD. Older persons may be at greatest risk of adverse sequelae due to the age-related decline in kidney function and lesser ability than young individuals to excrete an acid load [2–4]. This may have important consequences as alkali supplementation in postmenopausal women without overt acidosis has been shown to improve nitrogen balance and skeletal metabolism [5].

Changes in Muscle Physiology Due to Metabolic Acidosis

In otherwise healthy humans, there is a continuous cycle of muscle protein synthesis and degradation. This turnover is tightly regulated because even a minimal decrease in synthesis or increase in degradation can result in a net loss in muscle mass over time [6, 7]. Chronic metabolic acidosis disturbs this homeostasis, primarily by stimulating skeletal muscle protein breakdown. Acidosis also promotes amino acid oxidation and may impair muscle protein synthesis as well [8–11].

Three main systems have been described in muscle protein degradation: lysosomal proteases (cathepsin system), the calcium-dependent calpain system, and the ATP-dependent ubiquitin-proteasome system (UPS) [12, 13]. Inhibition of the first two systems does not substantially suppress proteolysis in animal models of catabolic conditions [14, 15]. Therefore, quantitatively the UPS is the major pathway responsible for muscle protein degradation [16]. However, the UPS cannot degrade the complex structure of actomyosin. Caspase-3 initiates the process of protein degradation by catalyzing the disassembly of myofibrils into a characteristic 14-kDa actin fragment and other substrates that are then degraded by the UPS [17]. After activation by a ubiquitin activating enzyme, E1, ubiquitin moieties are transferred to an E2 carrier protein and then conjugated to the protein substrate complex by an E3 ubiquitin-protein ligase. This process of ubiquitination targets the protein for degradation by the proteasome. The E3 ligases are specific in their actions because they only recognize a limited range of target proteins. The muscle-specific E3 ligases, atrogin-1/muscle atrophy F-box (MAFbx) and muscle ring finger 1 (MuRF1), have been linked with muscle atrophy in CKD and other catabolic states [18–21].

A number of factors stimulate muscle breakdown through the UPS [19, 22]. In addition to acidosis, these include catabolic states such as uremia, and factors including inflammation, angiotensin II, and disturbances in insulin and insulin-like growth factor-1 (IGF-1) function. Binding of insulin and IGF-1 to their respective receptors results in tyrosine phosphorylation of insulin receptor substrate (IRS) proteins. The phosphorylated IRS protein then serves as a recruitment site for phosphatidylinositol 3-kinase (PI3-K), which signals the downstream effector Akt. Downstream effects of PI3-K/Akt signaling simultaneously suppress catabolic pathways and promote muscle protein synthesis, thereby preventing muscle atrophy [18].

Metabolic acidosis suppresses the effects of this IRS/PI3-K/Akt pathway (Fig. 10.1) [23]. In a rat model of uremia, basal signaling through the PI3-K/Akt pathway in skeletal muscle was suppressed when compared to control animals. Normalization of the extracellular pH with a sodium bicarbonate-supplemented diet partially restored basal IRS-1 associated PI3-K activity and partially reversed the increase in muscle protein degradation [24]. Acidosis also augments the transcription of genes that code for the UPS [25]. Thus acidosis increases skeletal muscle proteolysis by suppressing IRS-1/PI3-K/Akt signaling, leading to activation of caspase-3 and the UPS. This clearly implicates metabolic acidosis as an important contributor to muscle proteolysis in CKD.

Alterations in Lean Mass and Muscle Function Due to Metabolic Acidosis

A number of studies in humans suggest that the treatment of acidosis ameliorates the insulin signaling defect in skeletal muscle and decreases muscle breakdown (Tables 10.1, 10.2, and 10.3). DeFronzo and Beckles induced insulin resistance in normal subjects by acidification with ammonium chloride, a model of chronic acidosis [26]. The defect was most likely due to an effect on skeletal muscle insulin sensitivity. Mak treated eight young subjects (mean age 18 years) receiving maintenance hemodialysis with oral sodium bicarbonate for 2 weeks and found an improvement in insulin sensitivity [27]. Reaich et al. treated eight patients with advanced CKD (mean serum creatinine 7.4 mg/dL) with oral sodium bicarbonate for 4 weeks and found improvements in insulin sensitivity and reduced whole-body protein breakdown [28]. Several studies in patients receiving peritoneal dialysis (PD) and maintenance hemodialysis have shown that correcting acidosis in end-stage renal disease patients reduces protein breakdown [29, 30]. Pickering et al. found a reduction in

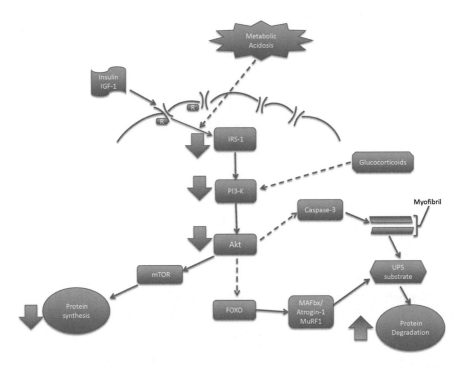

Fig. 10.1 Mechanism of metabolic acidosis-induced muscle protein breakdown. Acidosis (*bold arrows*) impairs signaling downstream of insulin and insulin-like growth factor-1 via the insulin receptor substrate/phosphatidylinositol 3-kinase/Akt pathway. This activates proteolytic pathways including caspase-3, which degrades actomyosin, producing substrates that are then degraded by the ubiquitin-proteasome system. Upregulation of FOXO stimulates expression of the E3 ubiquitin ligases MAFbx and MuRF1. Glucocorticoids appear to have a permissive effect on acidosis-induced proteolysis. Decreased activation of Akt may also impair protein synthesis by reducing mTOR activity. *Abbreviations*: *IGF-1* insulin-like growth factor-1, *IRS* insulin receptor substrate, *PI3-K* phosphatidylinositol 3-kinase, *UPS* ubiquitin-proteasome system, *MAFbx* muscle atrophy F-box, *MuRF1* muscle ring finger 1, *mTOR* mammalian target of rapamycin. "R" denotes insulin and IGF-1 receptors

skeletal muscle ubiquitin mRNA after correction of acidosis in eight PD patients, indicating that UPS-mediated proteolysis is ameliorated by alkali therapy [31]. Even a mild decrease in extracellular pH is sufficient to activate proteolysis. Ammonium chloride-induced acidosis in normal participants lowered pH from 7.42 to 7.35 and stimulated muscle protein degradation [32]. Furthermore, in healthy postmenopausal women without overt acidosis or CKD, oral potassium bicarbonate reduced urinary nitrogen excretion, suggesting an improvement in muscle protein breakdown [33].

Studies in patients with CKD with reduced GFR suggest that correction of acidosis also preserves muscle mass (Tables 10.1, 10.2, and 10.3). In a year-long single-blinded randomized trial of high versus low-alkali dialysate in 200 patients receiving PD, the high-alkali intervention led to weight gain, increased muscle mass (measured anthropometrically by mid-arm circumference), and fewer hospitalizations [34]. Of note, the difference in acid–base status between the two groups was relatively modest: at the end of the study, the mean pH and serum bicarbonate were

7.44 and 27.2 mEq/L in the high-alkali group and 7.40 and 23.0 mEq/L in the low-alkali group, respectively. Similarly, a double-blinded randomized trial of oral sodium bicarbonate in 60 PD patients found greater lean mass, higher Subjective Global Assessment scores (a nutritional assessment that includes muscle mass), and fewer days of hospitalization after 1 year [35]. Treatment with oral sodium bicar-

Table 10.1 Studies examining effects of metabolic acidosis on skeletal muscle in persons without kidney disease

Physiological studies/body composition	Outcome
Nitrogen balance before and after treatment of acidosis	$KHCO_3$ improved nitrogen balance [33, 48].
Protein breakdown and nitrogen balance before and after inducing acidosis	NH_4Cl increases protein breakdown [32] and induces negative nitrogen balance [10].
Amino acid oxidation before and after acidosis	NH_4Cl increases amino acid oxidation [32].
Albumin synthesis before and after inducing acidosis	Chronic NH_4Cl decreases albumin synthesis [10]. Acute NH_4Cl does not decrease albumin synthesis [49].
Muscle protein synthesis before and after inducing acidosis	Acute NH_4Cl decreases muscle protein synthesis [49].
Muscle strength and function	
Muscle performance before and after treatment with bicarbonate	Bicarbonate improved muscle performance in women but not in men [43].
Interval training before and after bicarbonate ingestion	$NaHCO_3$ improves endurance performance [38].
High intensity work before and after treatment of acidosis	$NaHCO_3$ improved performance in high intensity work [50].

Table 10.2 Studies examining effects of metabolic acidosis on skeletal muscle in persons with pre-dialysis chronic kidney disease

Physiological studies/body composition	Outcome
Skeletal muscle ubiquitin gene expression before and after sodium bicarbonate treatment	No difference in expression of ubiquitin mRNA with $NaHCO_3$ treatment [51].
Protein degradation and nitrogen balance before and after acidosis treatment	$NaHCO_3$ decreases protein degradation [9] and protein catabolic rate [52] and improves nitrogen balance [53].
Amino acid oxidation before and after treatment	$NaHCO_3$ decreases amino acid oxidation [9].
Serum albumin before and after acidosis treatment	Correction of acidosis improves serum albumin [36, 52].
Dietary protein intake and mid-arm muscle circumference before and after acidosis treatment	$NaHCO_3$ supplementation improves dietary protein intake and mid-arm muscle circumference and slows CKD progression [36].
Muscle strength and function	
Lower extremity muscle strength before and after acidosis treatment	$NaHCO_3$ treatment improved lower extremity muscle strength [42].

Table 10.3 Studies examining effects of metabolic acidosis on skeletal muscle in persons with chronic kidney disease requiring dialysis

Physiological studies/body composition	Outcome
Skeletal muscle levels of ubiquitin mRNA before and after treatment of acidosis	Ubiquitin mRNA decreased significantly after correcting acidosis [31].
Protein degradation before and after treatment of acidosis	Bicarbonate therapy decreased protein degradation [8, 29, 54–56].
Amino acid oxidation before and after treatment of acidosis	NaHCO₃ reduces amino acid oxidation [55].
Serum albumin levels before and after treatment of acidosis	Oral NaHCO₃ treatment failed to improve serum albumin [57, 58]. Oral NaHCO₃ improves serum albumin in patients without inflammation [8].
Nutritional status before and after treatment of acidosis	NaHCO₃ therapy improves subjective global assessment (SGA) score [35]. Sodium citrate treatment improves growth hormone sensitivity [59].
Changes in body composition before and after treatment of acidosis	Acidosis treatment increases body mass index, but no significant change in mid-arm circumference [31]. Triceps skin-fold thickness increased with bicarbonate dialysis [60]. No increase in triceps skin-fold with correction of acidosis [31, 34]. Correcting acidosis improves muscle and weight gain [31, 34].

bonate for 2 years also improved mid-arm circumference and increased serum albumin in patients with stage 4 CKD [36].

The adverse effects of metabolic acidosis on muscle physiology and muscle mass imply that correcting chronic acidosis might improve muscle strength and function (Tables 10.1 and 10.2). Indeed, alkali administration suppresses exercise-induced acidosis [37] and has produced improvements in short-term endurance performance and lactate threshold [38]. Epidemiologic data support this hypothesis. Among older adults in the general US population, metabolic acidosis was associated with slower gait speed, lower quadriceps strength, and greater likelihood of self-reported disability [39]. Lower serum bicarbonate due to metabolic acidosis was also associated with low cardiorespiratory fitness in younger adults, possibly mediated by changes in lean body mass, supporting the hypothesis that metabolic acidosis causes functional impairment via effects on skeletal muscle [40]. In a prospective observational study of older adults with and without CKD, lower serum bicarbonate was associated with a higher risk of incident functional limitation [41]. To date, two interventional studies have examined this question. Oral sodium bicarbonate administered to 20 adults with CKD and mild acidosis produced a dose-dependent increase in serum bicarbonate and improved lower extremity muscle strength after 6 weeks of therapy [42]. In healthy adults ≥50 years of age, 3 months of oral bicarbonate improved muscle strength in women but not men [43].

A reasonable approach to treating metabolic acidosis in patients with CKD is to first repeat the measurement of the serum bicarbonate. In selected patients a blood gas should be checked to rule out a respiratory acid–base disorder (in stable outpatients, a venous blood gas will suffice). While the optimal pH and serum bicarbonate are not known, the National Kidney Foundation Kidney Disease Outcomes Quality Initiative guidelines recommend maintaining serum bicarbonate ≥ 22 mEq/L [44]. For patients with only mild acidosis (e.g., serum bicarbonate ≥ 20 mEq/L), a dietary intervention alone is an appropriate first step [45]. This should focus on increasing fruit and vegetable intake, which will not only reduce the dietary acid load and raise the serum bicarbonate, but bestow additional important health benefits such as weight loss and improved blood pressure control [46, 47]. Because of the increased potassium intake, this intervention is only appropriate for patients at low risk of hyperkalemia. If dietary modification is not successful, and for patients with more severe acidosis, oral alkali should be prescribed. This should usually be initiated at a low dose (e.g., sodium bicarbonate 650 mg twice daily—each 650 mg tablet provides 7.74 mEq alkali) to minimize side effects. The dose can then be titrated to achieve the desired level of serum bicarbonate.

Conclusions

Chronic metabolic acidosis has a number of negative effects on skeletal muscle. While the physiologic alterations have been well-documented, only a few studies have addressed functional outcomes. In the case presented, mild metabolic acidosis is likely associated with increased muscle protein degradation relative to synthesis. Treatment of acidosis could reverse this defect and might, over time, preserve lean mass and muscle strength in this patient at risk for functional decline. Given the mild degree of acidosis and absence of hyperkalemia, a dietary intervention would be an appropriate first step after confirming that the serum bicarbonate is low (choice B). A blood gas is likely not required based on the clinical history. If treatment with oral sodium bicarbonate was subsequently required, it would be prudent to begin with a low dose.

References

1. Carrero JJ, Chmielewski M, Axelsson J, Snaedal S, Heimburger O, Barany P, et al. Muscle atrophy, inflammation and clinical outcome in incident and prevalent dialysis patients. Clin Nutr. 2008;27(4):557–64.
2. Frassetto LA, Morris Jr RC, Sebastian A. Effect of age on blood acid–base composition in adult humans: role of age-related renal functional decline. Am J Physiol. 1996;271(6 Pt 2):F1114–22.
3. Amodu A, Abramowitz MK. Dietary acid, age, and serum bicarbonate levels among adults in the United States. Clin J Am Soc Nephrol. 2013;8(12):2034–42.

4. Berkemeyer S, Vormann J, Gunther AL, Rylander R, Frassetto LA, Remer T. Renal net acid excretion capacity is comparable in prepubescence, adolescence, and young adulthood but falls with aging. J Am Geriatr Soc. 2008;56(8):1442–8.
5. Sebastian A, Harris ST, Ottaway JH, Todd KM, Morris Jr RC. Improved mineral balance and skeletal metabolism in postmenopausal women treated with potassium bicarbonate. N Engl J Med. 1994;330(25):1776–81.
6. Ciechanover A. The ubiquitin-mediated proteolytic pathway: mechanisms of action and cellular physiology. Biol Chem Hoppe Seyler. 1994;375(9):565–81.
7. Coux O, Tanaka K, Goldberg AL. Structure and functions of the 20S and 26S proteasomes. Annu Rev Biochem. 1996;65:801–47.
8. Movilli E, Viola BF, Camerini C, Mazzola G, Cancarini GC. Correction of metabolic acidosis on serum albumin and protein catabolism in hemodialysis patients. J Ren Nutr. 2009;19(2):172–7.
9. Reaich D, Channon SM, Scrimgeour CM, Daley SE, Wilkinson R, Goodship TH. Correction of acidosis in humans with CRF decreases protein degradation and amino acid oxidation. Am J Physiol. 1993;265(2 Pt 1):E230–5.
10. Ballmer PE, McNurlan MA, Hulter HN, Anderson SE, Garlick PJ, Krapf R. Chronic metabolic acidosis decreases albumin synthesis and induces negative nitrogen balance in humans. J Clin Invest. 1995;95(1):39–45.
11. England BK, Chastain JL, Mitch WE. Abnormalities in protein synthesis and degradation induced by extracellular pH in BC3H1 myocytes. Am J Physiol. 1991;260(2 Pt 1):C277–82.
12. Raj DS, Dominic EA, Pai A, Osman F, Morgan M, Pickett G, et al. Skeletal muscle, cytokines, and oxidative stress in end-stage renal disease. Kidney Int. 2005;68(5):2338–44.
13. Raj DS, Sun Y, Tzamaloukas AH. Hypercatabolism in dialysis patients. Curr Opin Nephrol Hypertens. 2008;17(6):589–94.
14. Workeneh BT, Mitch WE. Review of muscle wasting associated with chronic kidney disease. Am J Clin Nutr. 2010;91(4):1128S–32.
15. Lowell BB, Ruderman NB, Goodman MN. Evidence that lysosomes are not involved in the degradation of myofibrillar proteins in rat skeletal muscle. Biochem J. 1986;234(1):237–40.
16. Ciechanover A. Intracellular protein degradation: from a vague idea through the lysosome and the ubiquitin-proteasome system and onto human diseases and drug targeting. Bioorg Med Chem. 2013;21(12):3400–10.
17. Rajan VR, Mitch WE. Muscle wasting in chronic kidney disease: the role of the ubiquitin proteasome system and its clinical impact. Pediatr Nephrol. 2008;23(4):527–35.
18. Stitt TN, Drujan D, Clarke BA, Panaro F, Timofeyva Y, Kline WO, et al. The IGF-1/PI3K/Akt pathway prevents expression of muscle atrophy-induced ubiquitin ligases by inhibiting FOXO transcription factors. Mol Cell. 2004;14(3):395–403.
19. Lee SW. Regulation of muscle protein degradation: coordinated control of apoptotic and ubiquitin-proteasome systems by phosphatidylinositol 3 kinase. J Am Soc Nephrol. 2004;15(6):1537–45.
20. Galasso G, De Rosa R, Piscione F, Iaccarino G, Vosa C, Sorriento D, et al. Myocardial expression of FOXO3a-Atrogin-1 pathway in human heart failure. Eur J Heart Fail. 2010;12(12):1290–6.
21. Sandri M, Sandri C, Gilbert A, Skurk C, Calabria E, Picard A, et al. Foxo transcription factors induce the atrophy-related ubiquitin ligase atrogin-1 and cause skeletal muscle atrophy. Cell. 2004;117(3):399–412.
22. Du J, Wang X, Miereles C, Bailey JL, Debigare R, Zheng B, et al. Activation of caspase-3 is an initial step triggering accelerated muscle proteolysis in catabolic conditions. J Clin Invest. 2004;113(1):115–23.
23. Franch HA, Raissi S, Wang X, Zheng B, Bailey JL, Price SR. Acidosis impairs insulin receptor substrate-1-associated phosphoinositide 3-kinase signaling in muscle cells: consequences on proteolysis. Am J Physiol Renal Physiol. 2004;287(4):F700–6.

24. Bailey JL, Zheng B, Hu Z, Price SR, Mitch WE. Chronic kidney disease causes defects in signaling through the insulin receptor substrate/phosphatidylinositol 3-kinase/Akt pathway: implications for muscle atrophy. J Am Soc Nephrol. 2006;17(5):1388–94.
25. Bailey JL, Wang X, England BK, Price SR, Ding X, Mitch WE. The acidosis of chronic renal failure activates muscle proteolysis in rats by augmenting transcription of genes encoding proteins of the ATP-dependent ubiquitin-proteasome pathway. J Clin Invest. 1996;97(6):1447–53.
26. DeFronzo RA, Beckles AD. Glucose intolerance following chronic metabolic acidosis in man. Am J Physiol. 1979;236(4):E328–34.
27. Mak RH. Effect of metabolic acidosis on insulin action and secretion in uremia. Kidney Int. 1998;54(2):603–7.
28. Reaich D, Graham KA, Channon SM, Hetherington C, Scrimgeour CM, Wilkinson R, et al. Insulin-mediated changes in PD and glucose uptake after correction of acidosis in humans with CRF. Am J Physiol. 1995;268(1 Pt 1):E121–6.
29. Graham KA, Reaich D, Channon SM, Downie S, Gilmour E, Passlick-Deetjen J, et al. Correction of acidosis in CAPD decreases whole body protein degradation. Kidney Int. 1996;49(5):1396–400.
30. Lim VS, Bier DM, Flanigan MJ, Sum-Ping ST. The effect of hemodialysis on protein metabolism. A leucine kinetic study. J Clin Invest. 1993;91(6):2429–36.
31. Pickering WP, Price SR, Bircher G, Marinovic AC, Mitch WE, Walls J. Nutrition in CAPD: serum bicarbonate and the ubiquitin-proteasome system in muscle. Kidney Int. 2002;61(4):1286–92.
32. Reaich D, Channon SM, Scrimgeour CM, Goodship TH. Ammonium chloride-induced acidosis increases protein breakdown and amino acid oxidation in humans. Am J Physiol. 1992;263(4 Pt 1):E735–9.
33. Frassetto L, Morris Jr RC, Sebastian A. Potassium bicarbonate reduces urinary nitrogen excretion in postmenopausal women. J Clin Endocrinol Metab. 1997;82(1):254–9.
34. Stein A, Moorhouse J, Iles-Smith H, Baker F, Johnstone J, James G, et al. Role of an improvement in acid–base status and nutrition in CAPD patients. Kidney Int. 1997;52(4):1089–95.
35. Szeto CC. Oral sodium bicarbonate for the treatment of metabolic acidosis in peritoneal dialysis patients: a randomized placebo-control trial. J Am Soc Nephrol. 2003;14(8):2119–26.
36. de Brito-Ashurst I, Varagunam M, Raftery MJ, Yaqoob MM. Bicarbonate supplementation slows progression of CKD and improves nutritional status. J Am Soc Nephrol. 2009;20(9):2075–84.
37. Street D, Nielsen JJ, Bangsbo J, Juel C. Metabolic alkalosis reduces exercise-induced acidosis and potassium accumulation in human skeletal muscle interstitium. J Physiol. 2005;566(Pt 2):481–9.
38. Edge J, Bishop D, Goodman C. Effects of chronic NaHCO₃ ingestion during interval training on changes to muscle buffer capacity, metabolism, and short-term endurance performance. J Appl Physiol. 2006;101(3):918–25.
39. Abramowitz MK, Hostetter TH, Melamed ML. Association of serum bicarbonate levels with gait speed and quadriceps strength in older adults. Am J Kidney Dis. 2011;58(1):29–38.
40. Abramowitz MK, Hostetter TH, Melamed ML. Lower serum bicarbonate and a higher anion gap are associated with lower cardiorespiratory fitness in young adults. Kidney Int. 2012;81(10):1033–42.
41. Yenchek R, Ix JH, Rifkin DE, Shlipak MG, Sarnak MJ, Garcia M, et al. Association of serum bicarbonate with incident functional limitation in older adults. Clin J Am Soc Nephrol. 2014;9(12):2111–6.
42. Abramowitz MK, Melamed ML, Bauer C, Raff AC, Hostetter TH. Effects of oral sodium bicarbonate in patients with CKD. Clin J Am Soc Nephrol. 2013;8(5):714–20.
43. Dawson-Hughes B, Castaneda-Sceppa C, Harris SS, Palermo NJ, Cloutier G, Ceglia L, et al. Impact of supplementation with bicarbonate on lower-extremity muscle performance in older men and women. Osteoporos Int. 2010;21(7):1171–9. A journal established as result of coop-

eration between the European Foundation for Osteoporosis and the National Osteoporosis Foundation of the USA.

44. K/DOQI clinical practice guidelines for chronic kidney disease: evaluation, classification, and stratification. Am J Kidney Dis. 2002;39(2 Suppl 1):S1–266.

45. Chen W, Abramowitz MK. Treatment of metabolic acidosis in patients with CKD. Am J Kidney Dis. 2014;63(2):311–7.

46. Goraya N, Simoni J, Jo C, Wesson DE. Dietary acid reduction with fruits and vegetables or bicarbonate attenuates kidney injury in patients with a moderately reduced glomerular filtration rate due to hypertensive nephropathy. Kidney Int. 2012;81(1):86–93.

47. Goraya N, Simoni J, Jo CH, Wesson DE. A comparison of treating metabolic acidosis in CKD stage 4 hypertensive kidney disease with fruits and vegetables or sodium bicarbonate. Clin J Am Soc Nephrol. 2013;8(3):371–81.

48. Ceglia L, Harris SS, Abrams SA, Rasmussen HM, Dallal GE, Dawson-Hughes B. Potassium bicarbonate attenuates the urinary nitrogen excretion that accompanies an increase in dietary protein and may promote calcium absorption. J Clin Endocrinol Metab. 2009;94(2):645–53.

49. Kleger GR, Turgay M, Imoberdorf R, McNurlan MA, Garlick PJ, Ballmer PE. Acute metabolic acidosis decreases muscle protein synthesis but not albumin synthesis in humans. Am J Kidney Dis. 2001;38(6):1199–207.

50. McNaughton L, Backx K, Palmer G, Strange N. Effects of chronic bicarbonate ingestion on the performance of high-intensity work. Eur J Appl Physiol Occup Physiol. 1999;80(4): 333–6.

51. Roberts RG, Redfern CP, Graham KA, Bartlett K, Wilkinson R, Goodship TH. Sodium bicarbonate treatment and ubiquitin gene expression in acidotic human subjects with chronic renal failure. Eur J Clin Invest. 2002;32(7):488–92.

52. Verove C, Maisonneuve N, El Azouzi A, Boldron A, Azar R. Effect of the correction of metabolic acidosis on nutritional status in elderly patients with chronic renal failure. J Ren Nutr. 2002;12(4):224–8.

53. Papadoyannakis NJ, Stefanidis CJ, McGeown M. The effect of the correction of metabolic acidosis on nitrogen and potassium balance of patients with chronic renal failure. Am J Clin Nutr. 1984;40(3):623–7.

54. Graham KA, Reaich D, Channon SM, Downie S, Goodship TH. Correction of acidosis in hemodialysis decreases whole-body protein degradation. J Am Soc Nephrol. 1997;8(4):632–7.

55. Lim VS, Yarasheski KE, Flanigan MJ. The effect of uraemia, acidosis, and dialysis treatment on protein metabolism: a longitudinal leucine kinetic study. Nephrol Dial Transplant. 1998;13(7):1723–30.

56. Lofberg E, Gutierrez A, Anderstam B, Wernerman J, Bergstrom J, Price SR, et al. Effect of bicarbonate on muscle protein in patients receiving hemodialysis. Am J Kidney Dis. 2006;48(3):419–29.

57. Bossola M, Giungi S, Tazza L, Luciani G. Long-term oral sodium bicarbonate supplementation does not improve serum albumin levels in hemodialysis patients. Nephron Clin Pract. 2007;106(1):c51–6.

58. Ruggieri F, Caso G, Wegmann M, McNurlan MA, Wahl C, Imoberdorf R, et al. Does increasing blood pH stimulate protein synthesis in dialysis patients? Nephron Clin Pract. 2009;112(4):c276–83.

59. Wiederkehr MR, Kalogiros J, Krapf R. Correction of metabolic acidosis improves thyroid and growth hormone axes in haemodialysis patients. Nephrol Dial Transplant. 2004;19(5):1190–7.

60. Williams AJ, Dittmer ID, McArley A, Clarke J. High bicarbonate dialysate in haemodialysis patients: effects on acidosis and nutritional status. Nephrol Dial Transplant. 1997;12(12): 2633–7.

Chapter 11
Metabolic Acidosis Effects on Bone and Its Metabolism

Donald E. Wesson

Case

A 66-year-old African American man with a long history of type 2 diabetic nephropathy has an estimated GFR by the Modification of Diet in Renal Disease formula of 26 ml/min/1.73 m^2. He has presented with symptoms of bone pain, mild forearm and upper extremity bone pain in response to deep palpation, and laboratory findings consistent with increased bone resorption. Imaging studies are consistent with decreased bone mineral content. His serum total CO_2 (bicarbonate) on his routine laboratory panel was 20 mM (normal 20–29 mM for the clinical laboratory) and his clinician confirmed with blood gases that the low bicarbonate was due to non-anion gap metabolic acidosis. Which of the following is the best option for managing his metabolic acidosis?

(a) No specific treatment for his metabolic acidosis
(b) Oral sodium-based alkali therapy (sodium bicarbonate or sodium citrate) to maintain his serum bicarbonate concentration within the normal range (e.g., 24–29 mM)
(c) Intravenous sodium bicarbonate now, followed by chronic oral sodium bicarbonate
(d) A low acid diet, e.g., one high in base-producing fruits and vegetables
(e) A protein-restricted diet

We will discuss what current data support is the best of the listed management options at the end of this chapter.

D.E. Wesson, M.D., M.B.A. (✉)
Baylor Scott and White Health, Department of Internal Medicine, Texas A&M Health Sciences Center College of Medicine, 2401 South 31st Street, Temple, TX 76508, USA
e-mail: dwesson@sw.org

© Springer Science+Business Media New York 2016
D.E. Wesson (ed.), *Metabolic Acidosis*, DOI 10.1007/978-1-4939-3463-8_11

Introduction

Some data support that dietary acid challenges to systemic acid–base balance have adverse effects on bone health, even in patients without baseline metabolic acidosis [1]. The key feature of these diets proposed to injure bone is that they contain high amounts of components, particularly animal-sourced protein, which increase net endogenous acid production [2, 3]. Such acid-producing diets cause only minor changes in plasma acid–base parameters, typically within normal ranges for these parameters, even when inducing large increases in urine net acid excretion [4]. Nevertheless, these acid-producing diets can cause urine biochemical changes consistent with increased bone resorption [5]. Relatedly, oral alkali to reduce the high acid-producing aspect typical of Western diets increased bone mineral density and microarchitecture in elderly adults at increased risk for, but who did not at the time of study have, osteoporosis [6]. In addition, oral alkali improved mineral balance and bone metabolism in elderly women with osteoporosis [7]. Although not all studies support a role for high dietary acid in osteoporosis or increased fracture risk for community-dwelling patients without baseline metabolic acidosis [8], this remains an active area of research given that osteoporosis is a major health challenge, particularly among the elderly [9].

Published data more consistently support that baseline chronic metabolic acidosis injures bone. Experimentally induced chronic metabolic acidosis in animals decreased bone mineral density [10] and chronic metabolic acidosis in patients is associated with bone loss [11, 12]. On the other hand, oral alkali correction of metabolic acidosis due to renal tubular acidosis in children improved bone growth, mineral density, and histopathology [13, 14]. In addition, improvement of metabolic acidosis in dialysis-dependent patients reduced bone resorption and improved bone formation [15, 16]. Because low plasma levels of vitamin D and high levels of parathyroid hormone (PTH) occur in patients with reduced GFR at levels that are well above those for which kidney-replacement therapy is needed [17] but in whom metabolic acidosis might be observed [18], studies are needed to determine if correction of chronic metabolic acidosis in non-dialysis-dependent chronic kidney disease (CKD) corrects the disturbed mineral metabolism in these patients.

Normal Bone Physiology and Homeostasis

Normal bone is about one-third by volume organic, unmineralized matrix called osteoid. It is comprised predominately by type 1 collagen and small amounts of proteoglycan, lipids, and several non-collagenous proteins [19]. The remaining two-thirds is inorganic mineral, most of which is hydroxyapatite crystal made up of calcium, phosphate, and other ions such as hydroxyl and carbonate. The skeleton contains 80 % of body carbonate and 80 % of body citrate, each of which are potential buffers of H^+ [19]. The large surface area of bone makes these and other mineral constituents that can buffer H^+, like phosphate, readily available to buffer H^+ formed through metabolic processes, including dietary components that yield H^+ when metabolized.

Bone mass continuously turns over during life through a well-regulated coupling of bone formation and resorption [19]. During growth, bone formation exceeds resorption but after bone mass peaks at about ages 20–30 years, formation equals resorption [19]. After age 40–50 years, resorption exceeds formation by amounts that vary among individuals for reasons that have not been clearly elucidated. Two cell types are largely responsible for this resorption/formation process known as remodeling: osteoblasts are generally responsible for bone formation and osteoclasts are responsible for bone resorption.

Acid–Base Effects on Bone-Related Mineral Homeostasis

Calcium

Most (99 %) body calcium is in the skeleton with the remaining 1 % in extracellular and intracellular spaces. About 1 % of skeletal calcium is freely exchangeable with calcium in the extracellular fluid (ECF). Serum calcium is in three components: ionized, protein-bound, and complexed to divalent anions. The ionized fraction is typically ~48 % of the serum total [20] in the absence of changes from normal acid–base status. Protein-bound (mostly to albumin) calcium is typically ~46 % of the serum total [20] but because hydrogen ions compete with calcium for binding to albumin, an increase in serum hydrogen ion concentration (acidemia) as might occur with acidosis, reduces the protein-bound component and correspondingly increases the ionized component. The complexed component is ~7 % of total serum calcium [20].

Net gastrointestinal tract absorption is about 20 % of dietary calcium and most of that is from the small bowel, particularly the ileum. Healthy adults with steady-state bone mineral content excrete all the calcium absorbed from the gastrointestinal tract [20]. Individuals ingesting diets high in animal-sourced protein have increased urine calcium excretion [11, 21–24]. Earlier studies supported that this increased urine calcium excretion was due to bone buffering of acid produced from metabolism of the ingested animal protein with resorption of bone mineral and release of calcium into ECF [11, 21, 22]. More recent studies support that a likely greater contributor to the increased urine calcium excretion observed with these diets high in animal-sourced protein is that such diets are typically very low in oxalate that binds to calcium in the gut, thereby preventing calcium absorption and promoting fecal excretion. Greater gastrointestinal calcium absorption promoted by these low oxalate diets leads to increased urine calcium excretion [23, 24]. On the other hand, diets high in plant-sourced protein have high amounts of calcium-binding oxalate that yield decreased gastrointestinal calcium absorption with subsequent decreased urine calcium excretion [23, 24].

Phosphorous

Like calcium, most body phosphorous is in the skeleton with <1 % being in serum and most of that as phosphate. Phosphate absorbed from the gastrointestinal tract is transported into cells, deposited into bone or soft tissue, or eliminated from the body, mostly by the kidneys in the urine [20]. Serum alkalemia drives phosphate intracellularly, promoting hypophosphatemia while acidemia associated with acidosis has the opposite effect.

Dietary phosphate is absorbed predominantly in the stomach and upper small bowel with progressively less reabsorption as dietary contents move from the duodenum to the ileum. Diets high in animal-sourced protein tend also to be high in phosphorous and low in food components like grains and other plant-based proteins that contain phosphate-binding phytates which limit gastrointestinal phosphate absorption [25, 26]. Limiting dietary intake of phosphate, and importantly, limiting its gastrointestinal absorption, appears important to bone health because its increased intake is associated with increased risk of fractures in community-dwelling adults [27]. Conversely, diets in which protein intake is predominantly plant-based yield less gastrointestinal phosphate absorption and less urine phosphate excretion [25, 26]. Metabolic acidosis increases urine phosphate excretion, contributing to the component of urine acid excretion known as titratable acidity [28].

Magnesium

Similar to what has been described for calcium and phosphorous, most (99 %) of body magnesium is intracellular and most of this is in bone (60 %), muscle and soft tissue (25 %), with only 1 % being in ECF [29]. Sixty percent of serum magnesium is ionized, 30 % is bound to albumin, and 10 % is complexed to serum divalent anions [30]. Most dietary magnesium is absorbed in the small bowel with smaller amounts in the colon [20]. Increases in dietary magnesium decrease the percentage of gastrointestinal magnesium reabsorption and vice versa [31]. Metabolic acidosis decreases kidney magnesium reabsorption and thereby increases urine magnesium excretion [20].

Metabolic Acidosis Effects on Bone Physiology

Proton (H^+)-Induced Bone Dissolution

Experimental studies in vitro support that acute increases in extracellular [H^+] (decrease in pH) promote calcium release from bone directly through physical/chemical mechanisms without participation of cells [32, 33]. By contrast, calcium release from bone induced by chronic metabolic acidosis required the presence of live cells, notably osteoclasts [34, 35]. In vivo animal studies showed that acute metabolic acidosis increased serum calcium in the absence of PTH and inhibitors of bone cell action [36]. Because of the greater prevalence and duration of chronic metabolic acidosis compared to the acute variety, the chronic variety likely contributes most to the adverse consequences on bone by metabolic acidosis.

Metabolic acidosis commonly accompanies CKD [37, 38] and increases ECF free H^+ concentration (increased $[H^+]$ = decreased ECF pH). Part of body defenses to limit the untoward effects of free H^+ on tissues is to bind some of the free H^+ to various buffers. Bone serves as an important H^+ buffer system that minimizes the rise in ECF $[H^+]$ that might otherwise occur with chronic metabolic acidosis in CKD [19, 21]. In vivo studies show that bone incubated in acid media takes up H^+ in exchange for bone Na^+ and K^+ and that the media become more alkaline, consistent with release of base equivalents [39]. This release of bone base equivalents was supported by further studies directly showing depletion of bone carbonate stores in intact animals with chronic metabolic acidosis [40] and by in vivo bone studies showing release of calcium and carbonate from bone incubated in acid media [41]. The process leads to the short-term physiological benefit of H^+-buffering to limit its untoward effects on other tissues as described but also leads to the long-term pathophysiologic consequence of bone dissolution.

Increased Osteoclast-Mediated Bone Resorption

In addition to the physiochemical effects of increased $[H^+]$ on bone content described, increased $[H^+]$ increases activities of bone cells that increase bone resorption. Osteoclast H^+ secretion is an important component of the process by which osteoclasts resorb bone and this H^+ secretion is enhanced in cells incubated in acid media [42]. This increased bone resorption is part of the normal process of continuously replacing mineral in normal bone with new mineral. Ordinarily, this mineral resorption is quickly followed by mineral replacement in individuals with good bone health such that overall total mineral content of bone remains constant. This is not the circumstance with chronic metabolic acidosis, best described with CKD, which will be discussed subsequently. Increased bone resorption by osteoclasts in this setting of increased serum $[H^+]$ is enhanced by PTH [43].

Inhibition of Osteoblast-Mediated Bone Formation

Metabolic acidosis directly suppresses osteoblastic-induced collagen formation [44] thereby reducing new bone formation. Studies in experimental animals showed that chronic metabolic acidosis enhanced bone resorption and impaired bone formation [43]. This combination of increased bone resorption described earlier and decreased bone formation leads to increased urine calcium excretion and to total body negative calcium balance in CKD patients [45]. The combination of increased osteoclast activity with increased bone resorption and decreased osteoblast activity with decreased bone formation that characterizes chronic metabolic acidosis in CKD contributes to the syndrome known as renal or kidney osteodystrophy in CKD [46].

H+-Induced Alteration of Serum Concentrations and/or Biological Actions of PTH and Vitamin D

The calcemic response of bone to PTH is enhanced in the presence of metabolic acidosis [47] possibly mediated by enhanced uptake of PTH by bone cells and by enhanced PTH-mediated cyclic AMP production [48]. Metabolic acidosis in kidney failure reduces vitamin D production in animals [49] and alkali correction of metabolic acidosis in patients with kidney failure increases serum 1, 25 OH-vitamin D levels despite experimentally maintained serum levels of ionized calcium concentration and no changes in serum levels of magnesium, phosphate, albumin, or 25-OH-vitamin D [50]. Nevertheless, the serum level of the active form of vitamin D (1, 25, OH-vitamin D) in patients without CKD undergoing 9 days of metabolic acidosis induced by oral NH_4Cl was not different from control and its increase in response to infused PTH was also not different [51]. On the other hand, serum levels of the active form of vitamin D decreased as creatinine clearance decreased [52]. Together, the data support that metabolic acidosis is not a major contributor to the disturbed vitamin D metabolism of CKD.

Metabolic Acidosis Possibly Contributes to Fracture Risk in CKD

As indicated, metabolic acidosis contributes to the disturbed bone metabolism of CKD [46], is more likely in subjects with reduced compared to normal GFR, and metabolic acidosis is more severe in subjects with lower compared to higher levels of GFR [38]. This association might help explain why fracture risk among community-dwelling adults was higher in those with reduced compared to normal GFR [53]. For older women, a group at particularly high risk for hip fracture, there was a progressive inverse association between GFR and hip fracture in these women who were otherwise healthy [54]. Similar findings were reported for older women with regard to hip but not vertebral fractures [55]. This increased hip fracture risk for patients with reduced GFR was independent of traditional risk factors including age, body weight, and bone density. By contrast, the risk for vertebral fractures in this cohort was related to more traditional risk factors for fracture in this group such as older age and low bone mineral density [55]. Other studies report that reduced kidney function was particularly associated with increased fracture risk in younger (age 50–74 years) than older (>74 years) and that the risk was higher in those with severe compared to moderate reductions in GFR [56]. Furthermore, the 3-year cross-sectional risk of fracture for community-dwelling men and women >40 years of age increased in a graded fashion as GFR decreased [57]. Elucidation of the reasons why CKD is more strongly associated with fracture risk in hip compared to vertebral fractures and in younger compared to older individuals will require further study.

Conclusions

In vitro, in vivo laboratory data, and clinical data support that acid challenges to systemic acid–base status adversely affect bone metabolism. Although some data suggest that high acid-producing diets without metabolic acidosis can cause bone injury sufficient to yield adverse clinical outcomes, the data are more consistent that chronic metabolic acidosis, particularly in association with CKD, causes clinically significant bone injury. In addition, epidemiologic studies strongly associate CKD and its severity with increased fracture risk. Because of the association of metabolic acidosis with CKD and the severity of CKD, these data support an important contribution of the metabolic acidosis of CKD to the increased fracture rates suffered by these patients. Unfortunately, few published studies have examined the potential benefit of correction of metabolic acidosis upon this increased fracture risk. Until such studies are done, it seems prudent for clinicians to follow current guidelines that recommend alkali treatment of metabolic acidosis associated with CKD when serum total CO_2 is <22 mM [58].

Returning to the Case

The research that will yield a definitive answer to this case question is still evolving. Nevertheless, the most recent guidelines for treatment of metabolic acidosis in CKD recommend treating patients whose total CO_2 is <22 mM with oral, sodium-based alkali (sodium bicarbonate or sodium citrate) to maintain serum total CO_2 in a normal range [58]. Because this recommendation is based on opinion but limited clinical data, ongoing clinical studies will help determine if this recommendation should be modified. Consequently, selection "a" is contrary to this recommendation and selection "b" is the recommendation itself. Because the metabolic acidosis is mild as typically is the case with CKD, there is no urgency to treat the patient with intravenous bicarbonate so selection "c" is not the best choice. Some recent studies show that base-inducing fruits and vegetables can increase serum TCO_2 in CKD patients with metabolic acidosis [59, 60] but there are no published studies supporting that this treatment improves metabolic bone disease in CKD. In addition, such diets increase dietary potassium and CKD patients with eGFR as low as in our patient are at increased risk for hyperkalemia. Consequently, selection "d" is not the best choice. Diets high in animal-sourced protein might be expected to worsen existing metabolic acidosis. Those high in plant-sourced protein might improve metabolic acidosis if they are base-producing proteins but as stated, such diets have not been shown to improve the metabolic bone disease of CKD so "e" is not the best choice.

References

1. Pizzorno J, Frassetto LA, Katzinger J. Diet-induced acidosis: is it real and clinically relevant? Br J Nutr. 2010;103:1185–94.
2. Frassetto LA, Todd KM, Morris Jr RC, Sebastian A. Estimation of net endogenous noncarbonic acid production in humans from diet potassium and protein contents. Am J Clin Nutr. 1998;68:576–83.
3. Frassetto LA, Lanham-New SA, MacDonald HM, Remer T, Sebastian A, Tucker KL, Tylavsky FA. Standardizing terminology for estimating the diet-dependent net acid load to the metabolic system. J Nutr. 2007;137:1491–2.
4. Kurtz I, Maher T, Hulter HN, Schambelan M, Sebastian A. Effect of diet on plasma acid–base composition in normal humans. Kidney Int. 1983;24:670–80.
5. Buclin T, Cosma M, Appenzeller M, Jacquet AF, Decosterd LA, Biollaz J, Burckhardt P. Diet acids and alkalis influence calcium retention in bone. Osteoporos Int. 2001;12:493–9.
6. Jehle S, Hulter HN, Krapf R. Effect of potassium citrate on bone density, microarchitecture, and fracture risk in healthy older adults without osteoporosis: a randomized controlled trial. J Clin Endocrinol Metab. 2013;98:207–17.
7. Sebastian A, Harris ST, Ottaway JH, Todd KM, Morris Jr RC. Improved mineral balance and skeletal metabolism in postmenopausal women treated with potassium bicarbonate. N Engl J Med. 1994;330:1776–81.
8. Jia T, Byberg L, Lindhom B, Larsson TE, Lind L, Michaelsson K, Carrero JJ. Dietary acid load, kidney, function, osteoporosis, and risk of fractures in elderly men and women. Osteoporos Int. 2015;26:563–70.
9. Burge R, Dawson-Hughes B, Solomon DH, Wong JB, King A, Toteson A. Incidence and economic burden of osteoporosis-related fractures in the United States. J Bone Miner Res. 2007;22:465–75.
10. MacLeay JM, Olsen JD, Ennus RM, Les CM, Toth CA, Wheeler KL, Turner DL. Dietary-induced metabolic acidosis decreases bone mineral density in mature ovariectomized ewes. Calcif Tissue Int. 2004;75:431–7.
11. Lemann Jr J, Litzow JR, Lennon EJ. Studies of the mechanism by which chronic metabolic acidosis augments urinary calcium excretion in man. J Clin Invest. 1967;46:1318–28.
12. Mitch WE. Metabolic and clinical consequences of metabolic acidosis. J Nephrol. 2006;19 Suppl 9:S70–5.
13. McSherry E, Morris Jr RC. Attainment and maintenance of normal stature with alkali therapy in infants and children with classic renal tubular acidosis. J Clin Invest. 1978;61:509–27.
14. Domrongkitchaiporn S, Pongskul C, Sirikulchayanonta V, et al. Bone histology and bone mineral density after correction of acidosis in distal renal tubule acidosis. Kidney Int. 2002;62:2160–6.
15. Lefebvre A, DeVernejoul MC, Gueris J, Goldfarb B, Graulet AM, Morieux C. Optimal correction of acidosis in hemodialysis changes progression of dialysis osteodystrophy. Kidney Int. 1989;36:1112–8.
16. Bushinsky DA. Nephrology forum: the contribution of acidosis to renal osteodystrophy. Kidney Int. 1999;47:1816–32.
17. Levin A, Bakris GL, Molitch M, Smulders M, Tain J, Williams LA, Andress DL. Prevalence of abnormal serum vitamin D, PTH, calcium, and phosphorous in patients with chronic kidney disease: results of the study to evaluate early kidney disease. Kidney Int. 2007;71:31–8.

18. Widmer B, Gerhardt RE, Harrington JT, Cohen JJ. Serum electrolytes and acid base composition: the influence of graded degrees of chronic renal failure. Arch Intern Med. 1979;139:1099–102.
19. Green J, Kleeman CR. Role of bone in regulation of systemic acid–base balance. Kidney Int. 1991;39:9–26.
20. Blaine J, Chonchol M, Levi M. Renal control of calcium, phosphate, and magnesium homeostasis. Clin J Am Soc Nephrol. 2014;10:1257–72. doi:10.2215/CJN.09750913.
21. Lemann Jr J, Bushinsky DA, Hamm LL. Bone buffering of acid and base in humans. Am J Physiol. 2003;285:F811–32.
22. Goodman AD, Lemann C, Lennon EJ, et al. Production, excretion and net balance of fixed acids in patients with renal acidosis. J Clin Invest. 1965;44:495–506.
23. Cao JJ, Nielsen FH. Acid diet (high meat protein) effects on calcium metabolism and bone health. Curr Opin Clin Nutr Metab Care. 2010;13:698–702.
24. Cao JJ, Johnson LK, Hunt JR. A diet high in meat protein and potential renal acid load increases fractional calcium absorption and urinary calcium excretion without affecting markers of bone resorption or formation in postmenopausal women. J Nutr. 2011;141:391–7.
25. Moe SM, Zidehsarai MP, Chambers MA, Jackman LA, Radcliffe JS, Trevino LL, Donahue SE, Asplin JR. Vegetarian compared with meat dietary protein source and phosphorous homeostasis in chronic kidney disease. Clin J Am Soc Nephrol. 2011;6:257–64.
26. Moorthi RN, Armstrong CLH, Janda K, Ponsler-Sipes K, Asplin JR, Moe SM. The effect of a diet containing 70% protein from plants on mineral metabolism and musculoskeletal health in chronic kidney disease. Am J Nephrol. 2014;40:582–91.
27. Pinheiro MM, Schuch NJ, Gearo PS, Ciconelli RM, Ferraz MB, Martini A. Nutrient intakes related to osteoporotic fractures in men and women – the Brazilian Osteoporosis Study (BRAZOS). Nutr J. 2009;8:6. doi:10.1186/1475-2891-8-6.
28. Nowick M, Picard N, Stange G, Capuano P, Tenenhorse HS, Biber J, Murer H, Wagner CA. Renal phosphaturia during metabolic acidosis revisited: molecular mechanisms for decreased renal phosphate reabsorption. Pflugers Arch. 2008;457:539–49.
29. Konrad M, Schlingmann KP, Gudermann T. Insights into the molecular nature of magnesium homeostasis. Am J Physiol Renal Physiol. 2004;286:F599–605.
30. Sanders GT, Huijgen JG, Sanders R. Magnesium in disease: a review with special emphasis on the serum ionized magnesium. Clin Chem Lab Med. 1999;37:1011–33.
31. Fine KD, Santa Ana CA, Porter JL, Fordtran JS. Intestinal absorption of magnesium from food and supplements. J Clin Invest. 1991;88:396–402.
32. Dominguez JH, Raisz LG. Effects of changing hydrogen ion, carbonic acid and bicarbonate concentration on bone resorption in vitro. Calcif Tissue Int. 1979;29:7–13.
33. Bushinsky DA, Goldring JM, Coe FL. Cellular contribution to pH-mediated calcium flux in neonatal mouse calvariae. Am J Physiol. 1985;248:F785–9.
34. Bushinsky DA. Net calcium efflux from live bone during chronic metabolic but not respiratory acidosis. Am J Physiol. 1989;256:F836–42.
35. Goldhaber P, Rabadjija L. H+ stimulation of cell-mediated bone resorption in tissue culture. Am J Physiol. 1987;253:E90–8.
36. Kraut JA, Mishler DR, Kurokawa K. Effect of colchicine and calcitonin on calcemic response to metabolic acidosis. Kidney Int. 1984;30:608–12.
37. Relman AS. Renal acidosis and renal excretion of acid in health and disease. Adv Intern Med. 1964;12:295–347.
38. Hsu CY, Chertow GM. Elevations of serum phosphorous and potassium due to mild to moderate chronic renal insufficiency. Nephrol Dial Transplant. 2002;17:1419–25.
39. Bushinsky DA, Krieger NS, Geisser DI, et al. Effects of pH on bone calcium and proton fluxes in vivo. Am J Physiol. 1986;245:F204–9.
40. Bettice J. Skeletal carbon dioxide stores during metabolic acidosis. Am J Physiol. 1984;247:F326–30.
41. Bushinsky DA, Lechleider RJ. Mechanism of proton-induced calcium release: calcium carbonate dissolution. Am J Physiol. 1987;253:F998–1005.
42. Tett A, Blair HC, Schlesinger P, et al. Extracellular protons acidify osteoclasts, reduce cytosolic calcium and promote expression of cell-matrix attachment structures. J Clin Invest. 1989;84:773–81.

43. Kraut JA, Mishler DR, Singer FK, Goodman WG. The effects of metabolic acidosis on bone formation and bone resorption in the rat. Kidney Int. 1986;30:694–700.
44. Krieger NS, Sessler NE, Bushinsky DA. Acidosis inhibits osteoblastic and stimulates osteoclastic activity in vitro. Am J Physiol. 1992;262:F442–8.
45. Franch HA, Mitch WE. Catabolism in uremia: the impact of metabolic acidosis. J Am Soc Nephrol. 1998;9 Suppl 12:S78–81.
46. Kraut JA. The role of metabolic acidosis in the pathogenesis of renal osteodystrophy. Adv Ren Replace Ther. 1995;2:40–51.
47. Beck N, Webster SK. Effects of acute metabolic acidosis on parathyroid hormone action and calcium mobilization. Am J Physiol. 1976;230:127–31.
48. Martin KJ, Freitag JJ, Bellorin-Font E, et al. The effect of acute acidosis on the uptake of parathyroid hormone and the production of adenosine $3',5'$-monophosphate by isolated perfused bone. Endocrinology. 1980;106:1067–611.
49. Chan YL, Sardie E, Mason RS, Posen S. The effect of metabolic acidosis on vitamin D metabolism and bone histology in uremic rats. Calcif Tissue Int. 1985;37:158–64.
50. Lu K-C, Lin S-H, Yu F-C, Chyr SH, Shieh S-D. Influence of metabolic acidosis on serum 1, $25(OH)_2D_3$ levels in chronic renal failure. Miner Electrolyte Metab. 1985;21:398–402.
51. Kraut JA, Gordon EM, Ransom JC, Horst R, Slatopolsky E, Coburn JW, Kurokawa K. Effect of chronic metabolic acidosis on vitamin D metabolism in humans. Kidney Int. 1983;24:644–8.
52. Martinez I, Saracho R, Montenegro J, Lach F. The importance of dietary calcium and phosphorous in the secondary hyperparathyroidism of patients with early renal failure. Am J Kidney Dis. 1997;29:496–502.
53. Naylor KL, Garg AX, Zou G, Langsetmo L, Leslie WD, Fraser L-A, Adachi JD, Morin S, Goltzman D, Lentle B, Jackson SA, Josse RG, Jamal SA. Comparison of fracture risk prediction among individuals with reduced and normal kidney function. Clin J Am Soc Nephrol. 2015;10:646–53. doi:10.2215/CJN.06040614.
54. Fried LF, Biggs ML, Shlipak MG, Seiger S, Kestenbaum B, Stehman-Breen C, Sarnak M, Siscovick D, Harris T, Cauley J, Newman AB, Robbins J. Association of kidney function with incident hip fracture in older adults. J Am Soc Nephrol. 2007;18:282–6.
55. Ensrud KE, Lui L-Y, Taylor BC, Ishani A, Shlipak MG, Stone KL, Cauley JA, Jamal SA, Antoniucci DM, Cummings SR. Renal function in risk of hip and vertebral fractures in older women. Arch Intern Med. 2007;167:133–9.
56. Nickolas TL, McMahon DJ, Shane E. Relationship between moderate to severe kidney disease and hip fracture in the United States. J Am Soc Nephrol. 2006;17:3223–32.
57. Naylor KL, McArthur E, Leslie WD, Fraser L-A, Jamal SA, Cadarette SM, Pouget JG, Lok CE, Hodsman AB, Adachi JD, Garg AX. The three-year incidence of fracture in chronic kidney disease. Kidney Int. 2014;86:810–8.
58. National Kidney Foundation. K/DOQI clinical practice guidelines for nutrition in chronic renal failure. Am J Kidney Dis. 2000;35:S1–140.
59. Goraya N, Simoni J, Jo C-H, Wesson DE. Comparison of treating the metabolic acidosis of CKD stage 4 hypertensive kidney disease with fruits and vegetables or sodium bicarbonate. Clin J Am Soc Nephrol. 2013;8:371–81.
60. Goraya N, Simoni J, Jo C-H, Wesson DE. Treatment of metabolic acidosis in individuals with stage 3 CKD with fruits and vegetables or oral $NaHCO_3$ reduces urine angiotensinogen and preserves GFR. Kidney Int. 2014;86:1031–8.

Chapter 12
Endocrine Consequences of Metabolic Acidosis

Donald E. Wesson

Case

A 69-year-old African American man without a previous history of diabetes mellitus has been on three times weekly, 12-h/week, center-based hemodialysis for the past 3 years. He has had a progressive increase in fasting plasma blood glucose for the past year and his health care team is considering starting pharmacologic hypoglycemic therapy. His fasting plasma blood glucose improved only slightly in response to appropriate dietary instructions. In addition, as his residual kidney function has progressively decreased, his pre-dialysis plasma total CO_2 (HCO_3 concentration) has also progressively decreased with his most recent value being 16 mM. Which of the following is the best approach to treat his apparently worsening metabolic acidosis, particularly in light of the progressive increase in his fasting plasma glucose level?

(a) Increase the HCO_3 concentration in his dialysis bath above that of the standard bath against which he is currently being dialyzed
(b) Daily oral Na^+-based alkali therapy ($NaHCO_3$ or Na^+ citrate) to maintain his plasma bicarbonate concentration within the normal range (e.g., 24–29 mM)
(c) Pre-dialysis intravenous $NaHCO_3$ to increase his plasma HCO_3 concentration into the normal range (e.g., 24–29 mM) then complete his dialysis treatment as usual
(d) A low-acid diet, e.g., one high in base-producing fruits and vegetables
(e) No effort to increase his pre-dialysis plasma HCO_3 concentration

We will discuss what current data support is the best of the listed management options at the end of this chapter.

D.E. Wesson, M.D., M.B.A. (✉)
Baylor Scott and White Health, Department of Internal Medicine, Texas A&M Health Sciences Center College of Medicine, 2401 South 31st Street, Temple, TX 76508, USA
e-mail: dwesson@sw.org

© Springer Science+Business Media New York 2016
D.E. Wesson (ed.), *Metabolic Acidosis*, DOI 10.1007/978-1-4939-3463-8_12

Introduction

As detailed in other chapters of this book, metabolic acidosis is systemic process with adverse systemic consequences that are associated with increased mortality, even in patients whose reduced but remaining GFR is sufficient to not require kidney replacement therapy [1]. A possible contributor to the increased mortality associated with metabolic acidosis is increased risk for cardiovascular events [2]. The latter association assumes great importance recognizing that cardiovascular disease is in great excess among patients with chronic kidney disease (CKD) compared to similar patients without CKD [3]. Disturbances in endocrine physiology might contribute to some of the untoward outcomes associated with metabolic acidosis and this chapter will explore what is known about the pathophysiology of some of these endocrine disturbances. Because correction of metabolic acidosis is comparatively easy to accomplish, can be done with comparatively few side effects, and is comparatively inexpensive, studies are ongoing to determine if this intervention improves some of the untoward outcomes associated with metabolic acidosis.

Decreased Insulin Sensitivity (Increased Insulin Resistance)

Insulin resistance has been associated with the increased cardiovascular risk in dialysis-dependent CKD patients [4]. Nevertheless, insulin resistance appears early in the course of progressive decline in GFR, much before the need for kidney replacement therapy [5–8]. In pre-dialysis CKD patients, the degree of metabolic acidosis predicted the presence of insulin resistance and low serum bicarbonate was an independent contributing variable for insulin-mediated glucose disposal rate in CKD patients using stepwise multivariate regression analysis [8]. The latter data support a contributing role of metabolic acidosis in CKD to the observed insulin resistance. Earlier studies showed that patients without CKD and with baseline normal serum acid–base parameters developed insulin resistance when given NH_4Cl to induce chronic metabolic acidosis [9]. In addition, lower serum bicarbonate was associated with insulin resistance in patients in the National Health and Nutrition Examination Survey (NHANES) [10]. These data suggest that correction of metabolic acidosis improves insulin resistance but few published studies have tested this hypothesis. One such study in dialysis-dependent CKD patients showed that oral $NaHCO_3$ increased insulin sensitivity [11]. More studies testing this hypothesis in pre-dialysis CKD patients are very much needed, particularly in patients with reduced GFR but who do not require kidney replacement therapy like dialysis or kidney transplant.

Multiple mechanisms likely contribute to the impaired insulin sensitivity of chronic metabolic acidosis. Chronic metabolic acidosis decreases insulin sensitivity in experimental animals [12] mediated in part by reduced insulin binding to target sights in vitro [13]. Because infused angiotensin II induces insulin resistance in experimental animals [14] and metabolic acidosis activates the renin–angiotensin–aldosterone system (RAAS) in this same experimental model [15], metabolic acidosis-induced angiotensin II activity might contribute to insulin resistance. Oral NaHCO$_3$ reduces kidney angiotensin II levels augmented by acid retention in experimental animals with reduced GFR [16] so correction of metabolic acidosis in CKD patients might ameliorate the associated insulin resistance through reduction in kidney angiotensin II.

Disturbed Parathyroid Hormone and Vitamin D and Metabolism

Metabolic acidosis enhances the calcemic response of bone to PTH [17], possibly through augmented uptake of PTH by bone cells and by augmented PTH-mediated cyclic AMP production [18]. Metabolic acidosis in CKD reduces vitamin D production in experimental animals [19]. Alkali correction of metabolic acidosis in CKD increases serum 1, 25-OH vitamin D levels despite experimentally maintained serum levels of ionized calcium concentration and no changes in serum levels of magnesium, phosphate, albumin, or 25-OH vitamin D [20]. By contrast, serum levels of the active form of vitamin D (1, 25-OH vitamin D) were not different from control after 9 days of metabolic acidosis induced by oral NH$_4$Cl in patients without CKD [21]. Additionally, the PTH-induced increase in 1, 25-OH vitamin D was also not different [21] in these subjects with experimentally induced metabolic acidosis but without CKD [21]. On the other hand, serum levels of this active form of vitamin D decreased as creatinine clearance decreased [22]. These data support that metabolic acidosis itself is not a major contributor to the low serum levels of vitamin D in CKD patients with reduced GFR and that other factors more importantly contribute to decreased serum levels that commonly accompany reduced GFR.

Disturbed Glucocorticoid Metabolism

Chronic metabolic acidosis induced in humans with baseline normal kidney function with NH$_4$Cl increases glucocorticoid production leading to increased serum levels [23–25]. This increased glucocorticoid activity appears to convey the benefit of increased kidney acid excretion in the setting of metabolic acidosis [25] but also appears to contribute to adverse consequences associated with CKD such as disturbed bone [26] and muscle metabolism [27].

Disturbed Growth Hormone Metabolism

Patients with chronic metabolic acidosis have decreased sensitivity to growth hormone that leads to decreased levels of insulin growth factor-1 (IGF-1) [28, 29]. This insensitivity in hemodialysis-dependent CKD patients was improved by correction of their metabolic acidosis with oral Na^+ citrate [30]. Despite this relative insensitivity, administration of growth hormone to children with renal tubular acidosis reversed growth retardation due to the chronic metabolic acidosis [31]. In addition, growth hormone releasing hormone (GHRH) elicits an augmented increase in plasma levels of growth hormone in patients with chronic metabolic acidosis compared to individuals with normal acid–base status [29].

Disturbed Thyroid Hormone Metabolism

Experimentally produced chronic metabolic acidosis in humans caused mild hypothyroidism as manifest by significantly increased serum levels of thyroid stimulating hormone (TSH) with slight but significant decreases in serum levels of free T3 and free T4 [32]. These patients with experimentally induced metabolic acidosis also had an exaggerated response to thyrotropin (TRH) [32]. Although a comprehensive comparison of CKD patients with normal controls showed CKD patients with reduced serum levels of T3 and T4, they had normal TSH and a *blunted* response to TRH [33]. Together, these data suggest that although metabolic acidosis in CKD might contribute to some of its thyroid abnormalities, other CKD-related factors contribute to the disturbance in the pituitary/thyroid axis in CKD. In support of this, correction of metabolic acidosis in hemodialysis-dependent CKD patients with oral Na^+ citrate corrected serum free T3 levels but did not influence serum levels of free T4 or TSH [30]. Studies are needed to examine the effect of correction of metabolic acidosis in CKD patients with sufficient remaining GFR to not require kidney replacement therapy.

Alterations of the Renin–Angiotensin–Aldosterone System

Metabolic acidosis produced in experimental animals with NH_4Cl increased renin–angiotensin system activity [15]. In addition, experimental animals with the partial nephrectomy model of CKD have increased kidney levels of angiotensin II (AII) [16, 34] and aldosterone [35] that is mediated by acid retention associated with GFR reduction [16, 34, 35]. Furthermore, correction of acid retention related to reduce GFR with oral $NaHCO_3$ lowered kidney levels of AII [16, 34] and aldosterone [35].

Experimentally produced metabolic acidosis in patients increased activity of the RAAS [23, 24, 29]. In addition, patients with reduced GFR without metabolic acidosis but who appeared to have acid retention had increased plasma levels and urine excretion of aldosterone, each of which were reduced after oral $NaHCO_3$ [36]. Urine excretion of angiotensinogen reflects kidney levels of AII [37] and patients with reduced GFR and metabolic acidosis had increased urine excretion of angiotensinogen that was decreased after dietary acid reduction with $NaHCO_3$ or base-producing fruits and vegetables [38]. Because GFR decline in animal models of

CKD is mediated by AII [39] and/or through AII receptors [34] and because anti-AII drugs ameliorate GFR progression [40, 41], reduction of kidney AII activity by correction of metabolic acidosis might reduce untoward effects of high AII activities, possibly including nephropathy progression.

Altered Secretion of Catecholamines

Most studies examining the effect of metabolic acidosis on catecholamine release and serum levels have involved acute rather than chronic metabolic acidosis, and most such studies have examined this issue using animal models. Acute metabolic acidosis increased canine blood catecholamine levels [42] and in isolated canine adrenal glands [43]. In one of the few published human studies, acute metabolic acidosis induced by NH_4Cl infusions directly into the duodenum did not change plasma catecholamine levels hours later [44]. Whether longer exposure to the described metabolic acidosis affected plasma catecholamines was not examined by these investigators. Studies in humans examining the effects of chronic metabolic acidosis on plasma catecholamines, and its correction, are needed.

Stimulation of Kidney Endothelin Production

Animals with metabolic acidosis and reduced GFR had increased kidney levels of endothelin that decreased in response to oral $NaHCO_3$ [45]. Similarly, animals with reduced GFR without metabolic acidosis but with acid retention had high kidney endothelin levels that also decreased in response to dietary $NaHCO_3$ [35, 46]. In addition, increased dietary acid provided as mineral acid [47] or acid-producing dietary protein [48] increased kidney endothelin levels. Furthermore, an acid interstitial fluid environment of the kidney cortex in vivo is associated with reduced GFR and metabolic acidosis [45], is associated with reduced GFR without metabolic acidosis but with acid retention [35, 46], and is associated with increased dietary acid in animals with normal GFR [49]. Relatedly, decreased extracellular pH increased endothelin release from human kidney microvascular endothelial cells in vivo [50]. The latter studies suggest at least one cell source, microvascular endothelial cells, for the increase in kidney endothelin levels in response to an extracellular acid challenge. These data support an endothelin role to increase kidney acidification in the setting of reduced GFR and metabolic acidosis [45, 51], when GFR is reduced without metabolic acidosis but with acid retention [16], and in animals with normal baseline GFR in response to a dietary acid challenge provided by mineral acid [47] or acid-producing dietary protein [48].

Urine endothelin excretion is a surrogate for kidney endothelin levels [47] and urine endothelin excretion decreased in CKD patients with reduced GFR and metabolic acidosis in response to improvement of metabolic acidosis with oral Na^+

citrate [52]. In addition, CKD patients with reduced GFR without metabolic acidosis but with apparent acid retention had higher urine endothelin excretion than comparable patients with normal GFR [36]. Furthermore, dietary acid reduction done with oral $NaHCO_3$ reduced urine endothelin excretion in such patients [53], consistent with reduced urine endothelin levels [47]. Together, these data support that patients with metabolic acidosis associated with reduced GFR and those with reduced GFR without metabolic acidosis but with acid retention have increased kidney levels of endothelin.

Conclusions

Data to date show that metabolic acidosis, acid retention associated with reduced GFR but without metabolic acidosis, and increased dietary acid in subjects with normal baseline GFR and acid–base status can disturb multiple endocrine systems. These systemic consequences of acid challenges to systemic acid–base status have short-term and possibly long-term adverse consequences on endocrine systems. A few clinical studies show that correction of metabolic acidosis or amelioration of acid retention provides patient benefit but many more, larger, and longer term studies are needed to better determine the benefit, if any, on the endocrine disturbances associated with metabolic acidosis.

Returning to the Case

As with many aspects of the treatment of chronic metabolic acidosis, the research that will yield a definitive answer to this case question is still evolving. Few studies examining the potential benefits of correction of metabolic acidosis in patients with reduced GFR have been published. The most recent guidelines for treatment of metabolic acidosis in CKD recommend oral Na^+-based alkali ($NaHCO_3$ or Na^+ citrate) to maintain plasma total CO_2 in a normal range (24–29 mM) in patients with baseline total $CO_2 < 22$ mM [54]. A few published studies examined the benefit of improving metabolic acidosis in hemodialysis-dependent CKD patients. One showed that following this guideline in hemodialysis-dependent CKD to maintain pre-dialysis plasma total CO_2 at least 24 mM improved insulin sensitivity as measured by greater glucose disposal in response to insulin infusion [11]. Other investigators showed that treating hemodialysis-dependent CKD patients similarly improved sensitivity to growth hormone [30]. Consequently, selection "b" treatment with daily oral Na^+-based alkali to keep our patient's pre-dialysis plasma total CO_2 in the normal range is the option best supported by current data.

Published studies to date have not tested the approach indicated in selection "a" but this intervention to increase dialysate HCO_3 concentration in an effort to increase pre-dialysis plasma HCO_3 concentration did not reliably increase pre-dialysis plasma bicarbonate concentration [55] and is associated with increased mortality [56]. Selection "c" to infuse intravenous $NaHCO_3$ pre-dialysis to increase his plasma HCO_3 concentration into the normal range (e.g., 24–29 mM) also has not been examined in published studies. Nevertheless, having this done only once, three times weekly, is unlikely to dramatically increase plasma HCO_3 concentrations on non-dialysis days, something that would appear to be necessary to provide a sustained benefit on endocrine systems. The low-acid diet done with base-producing fruits and vegetables in selection "d" is an interesting approach that might have the same benefit as daily Na^+-based alkali therapy as it appears to have in small-scale studies that have been done examining the effect of dietary acid reduction on nephropathy progression [38]. This approach to improve insulin sensitivity in CKD patients with metabolic acidosis has yet to be tested in published studies, however. Because current guidelines recommend treatment of the metabolic acidosis of CKD patients with plasma total $CO_2 < 22$ mM with Na^+-based alkali, selection "e" that indicates no treatment for our patient's metabolic acidosis is not supported by current recommendations.

References

1. Kovesdy CP, Anderson JE, Kalantar-Zadeh K. Association of serum bicarbonate levels with mortality in patients with non-dialysis-dependent CKD. Nephrol Dial Transplant. 2009;24:1232–7.
2. Dobre M, Yang W, Chen J, Drawz P, Hamm LL, Horwitz E, et al. Association of serum bicarbonate with risk of renal and cardiovascular outcomes in CKD: a report from the Chronic Renal Insufficiency Cohort (CRIC) Study. Am J Kidney Dis. 2013;62:670–8.
3. Go AS, Chertow GM, Fan D, McCulloch CE, Hsu C-Y. Chronic kidney disease and the risk of death, cardiovascular events, and hospitalization. N Engl J Med. 2004;351:1296–305.
4. Shinohara K, Shoji Tm Emoto M, Tahara H, Koyama H, Ishimura E, Tabata T, Nishizawa Y. Insulin resistance as an independent predictor of cardiovascular mortality in patients with end-stage renal disease. J Am Soc Nephrol. 2002;13:1894–900.
5. Fliser D, Pacini G, Engelleiter R, Kautzky-Willer A, Franek I, Ritz E. Insulin resistance and hyperinsulinaemia are present already in patients with incipient renal disease. Kidney Int. 1998;53:1243–7.
6. Chen J, Muntner P, Hamm LL, Fonseca V, Batuman V, Whelton PK, He J. Insulin resistance and risk of chronic kidney disease in nondiabetic US adults. J Am Soc Nephrol. 2003;14:469–77.
7. Becker B, Kronenberg F, Kielstein JT, Haller H, Morath C, Ritz E, Fliser D. Renal insulin resistance syndrome, adiponectin, and cardiovascular events in patients with kidney disease: the mild and moderate kidney disease study. J Am Soc Nephrol. 2005;16:1091–8.
8. Kobayashi S, Maesato K, Moriya H, Ohtake T, Ikeda T. Insulin resistance in patients with chronic kidney disease. Am J Kidney Dis. 2005;45:275–80.
9. DeFronzo RA, Beckles AD. Glucose intolerance following chronic metabolic acidosis in man. Am J Physiol. 1979;236:E328–34.
10. Farwell WR, Taylor EN. Serum bicarbonate, anion gap, and insulin resistance in the National Health and Nutrition Examination Survey. Diabet Med. 2008;25:798–804.
11. Mak RH. Effect of metabolic acidosis on insulin action and secretion in uremia. Kidney Int. 1998;54:603–7.

12. Cuthbert C, Alberti KG. Acidemia and insulin resistance in diabetic ketoacidotic rat. Metabolism. 1978;27:1903–16.
13. Whittaker J, Cuthbert C, Hammond VA, Alberti KGM. The effects of metabolic acidosis in vivo on insulin binding to rat adipocytes. Metabolism. 1982;31:553–7.
14. Ogihara T, Asano T, Ando K, Chiba Y, Sakoda H, Anai M, Shojima N, Ono H, Onishi Y, Fujishiro M, Katagiri H, Fukusima Y, Kikuchi M, Noguchi N, Aburatani H, Kimuro I, Fujita T. Angiotensin II-induced insulin resistance is associated with enhanced insulin signaling. Hypertension. 2002;40:872–9.
15. Ng H-Y, Chen H-C, Tsai Y-C, et al. Activation of intrarenal renin-angiotensin system during metabolic acidosis. Am J Nephrol. 2011;34:55–63.
16. Wesson DE, Jo C-H, Simoni J. Angiotensin II receptors mediate increased distal nephron acidification caused by acid retention. Kidney Int. 2012;82:1184–94.
17. Beck N, Webster SK. Effects of acute metabolic acidosis on parathyroid hormone action and calcium mobilization. Am J Physiol. 1976;230:127–31.
18. Martin KJ, Freitag JJ, Bellorin-Font E, et al. The effect of acute acidosis on the uptake of parathyroid hormone and the production of adenosine 3′,5′-monophosphate by isolated perfused bone. Endocrinology. 1980;106:1067–611.
19. Chan YL, Sardie E, Mason RS, Posen S. The effect of metabolic acidosis on vitamin D metabolism and bone histology in uremic rats. Calcif Tissue Int. 1985;37:158–64.
20. Lu K-C, Lin S-H, Yu F-C, Chyr SH, Shieh S-D. Influence of metabolic acidosis on serum 1, 25(OH)$_2$D$_3$ levels in chronic renal failure. Miner Electrolyte Metab. 1985;21:398–402.
21. Kraut JA, Gordon EM, Ransom JC, Horst R, Slatopolsky E, Coburn JW, Kurokawa K. Effect of chronic metabolic acidosis on vitamin D metabolism in humans. Kidney Int. 1983;24:644–8.
22. Martinez I, Saracho R, Montenegro J, Lach F. The importance of dietary calcium and phosphorous in the secondary hyperparathyroidism of patients with early renal failure. Am J Kidney Dis. 1997;29:496–502.
23. Schambelan M, Sebastian A, Katuna A, Arteaga E. Adreno-cortical hormone secretory response to chronic NH$_4$Cl-induced metabolic acidosis. Am J Physiol. 1987;252:E454–60.
24. Henger A, Tutt P, Riesen WF, Hulter HN, Krapt R. Acid–base and endocrine effects of aldosterone and angiotensin II inhibition in metabolic acidosis in human patients. J Lab Clin Med. 2000;136:379–89.
25. Hulter HN, Licht JH, Bonner EL, Glynn RD, Sebastian A. Effects of glucocorticoid steroids on renal acid systemic acid–base metabolism. Am J Physiol. 1980;239:F30–43.
26. Kraut JA. The role of metabolic acidosis in the pathogenesis of renal osteodystrophy. Adv Ren Replace Ther. 1995;2:40–51.
27. May RC, Kelly RA, Mitch ME. Mechanisms for defects in muscle protein metabolism in rats with chronic uremia: the influence of metabolic acidosis. J Clin Invest. 1987;79:1099–103.
28. Brungger M, Hulter HN, Krapf R. Effect of chronic metabolic acidosis on the growth hormone/IGF-1 endocrine axis: new cause of growth hormone insensitivity in humans. Kidney Int. 1997;51:216–21.
29. Sicuro A, Mahlbacher K, Hulter HN, Krapf R. Effect of growth hormone on renal systemic acid–base homeostasis in humans. Am J Physiol. 1998;274:F650–7.
30. Wiederkehr MR, Kalogiros J, Krapf R. Correction of metabolic acidosis improves thyroid and growth hormone axes in hemodialysis patients. Nephrol Dial Transplant. 2004;19:1190–7.
31. McSherry E, Morris Jr RC. Attainment and maintenance of normal stature of alkali therapy in infants and children with classic renal tubular acidosis. J Clin Invest. 1978;61:509–27.
32. Brungger M, Hulter HN, Krapf R. Effect of chronic metabolic acidosis on thyroid hormone homeostasis in humans. Am J Physiol. 1997;272:F648–53.
33. Lim VS, Fang VS, Katz A, Refetoff S. Thyroid dysfunction in chronic renal failure. A study of the pituitary-thyroid axis and peripheral turnover kinetics of thyroxine and triiodothyronine. J Clin Invest. 1977;60:522–34.

34. Wesson DE, Jo C-H, Simoni J. Angiotensin II-mediated GFR decline in subtotal nephrectomy is due to acid retention associated with reduced GFR. Nephrol Dial Transplant. 2014;30:762–70. doi:10.1093/ndt/gfu388.

35. Wesson DE, Simoni J. Acid retention during kidney failure induces endothelin and aldosterone production which lead to progressive GFR decline, a situation ameliorated by alkali diet. Kidney Int. 2010;78:1128–35.

36. Wesson DE, Simoni J, Broglio K, Sheather S. Acid retention accompanies reduced GFR in humans and increases plasma levels of endothelin and aldosterone. Am J Physiol Renal Physiol. 2011;300:F830–7.

37. Kobori H, Harrison-Bernard LM, Navar G. Urinary excretion of angiotensinogen reflects intrarenal angiotensinogen production. Kidney Int. 2002;61:579–85.

38. Goraya N, Simoni J, Jo C-H, Wesson DE. Treatment of metabolic acidosis in individuals with stage 3 CKD with fruits and vegetables or oral NaHCO$_3$ reduces urine angiotensinogen and preserves GFR. Kidney Int. 2014;86:1031–8.

39. Anderson S, Rennke HG, Brenner BM. Therapeutic advantage of converting enzyme inhibitors in arresting progressive renal disease associated with systemic hypertension in the rat. J Clin Invest. 1986;77:1993–2000.

40. Lewis EJ, Hunsicker LC, Bain RP, Rohde RD and the Collaborative Study Group. The effect of angiotensin-converting enzyme inhibition on diabetic nephropathy. N Engl J Med. 1993;329:1456–62.

41. Wright JT, Bakris G, Greene T, Agodoa LY, Appel LJ, Charleston J. Effect of blood pressure lowering and antihypertensive drug class on progression of hypertensive kidney disease. JAMA. 2002;288:2421–31.

42. Morris ME, Millar RA. Blood pH/plasma catecholamine relationships: nonrespiratory acidosis. Br J Anaesth. 1962;34:682–9.

43. Nahas GFG, Zagury D, Milhaud A, Manger WM, Pappas GD. Acidemia and catecholamine output of the isolated canine adrenal gland. Am J Physiol. 1964;206:1281–4.

44. Wiederseiner J-M, Muser J, Lutz T, Hulter HN, Krapf R. Acute metabolic acidosis: characterization and diagnosis of the disorder and the plasma potassium response. J Am Soc Nephrol. 2004;15:1589–96.

45. Phisitkul S, Hacker C, Simoni J, Tran RM, Wesson DE. Dietary protein causes a decline in the glomerular filtration rate of the remnant kidney mediated by metabolic acidosis and endothelin receptors. Kidney Int. 2008;73:192–9.

46. Wesson DE, Simoni J. Increased tissue acid mediates progressive GFR decline in animals with reduced nephron mass. Kidney Int. 2009;75:929–35.

47. Wesson DE. Endogenous endothelins mediate increased distal tubule acidification induced by dietary acid in rats. J Clin Invest. 1997;99:2203–11.

48. Khanna A, Simoni J, Hacker C, Duran M-J, Wesson DE. Increased endothelin activity mediates augmented distal nephron acidification induced by dietary protein. J Am Soc Nephrol. 2004;15:2266–75.

49. Wesson DE. Dietary acid increases blood and renal cortical acid content in rats. Am J Physiol. 1998;274(Renal Physiol 43):F97–103.

50. Wesson DE, Simoni J, Green DF. Reduced extracellular pH increases endothelin-1 secretion by human renal microvascular cells. J Clin Invest. 1998;101:578–83.

51. Wesson DE. Endogenous endothelins mediate augmented acidification in remnant kidneys. J Am Soc Nephrol. 2001;12:1826–35.

52. Phisitkul S, Khanna A, Simoni J, Broglio K, Sheather S, Rajab H, Wesson DE. Amelioration of metabolic acidosis in subjects with low GFR reduces kidney endothelin production, reduces kidney injury, and better preserves GFR. Kidney Int. 2010;77:617–23.

53. Mahajan A, Simoni J, Sheather S, Broglio K, Rajab MH, Wesson DE. Daily oral sodium bicarbonate preserves glomerular filtration rate by slowing its decline in early hypertensive nephropathy. Kidney Int. 2010;78:303–9.

54. KDIGO Guidelines. Chapter 3: management of progression and complications of CKD. Kidney Int Suppl. 2013;3:73–90.

55. Noh US, Yi JH, Han SW, Kim HJ. Varying dialysate bicarbonate concentrations in hemodialysis patients affect post dialysis alkalosis but not pre-dialysis acidosis. Electrolyte Blood Press. 2007;5:95–101.
56. Tentori F, Karaboyas A, Robinson BM, Morgenstern H, Zhang J, Sen A, Ikizler TA, Rayner H, Fissell RB, Vanholder R, Tomo T, Port FK. Association of dialysate bicarbonate concentration with mortality in the Dialysis Outcomes and Practice Patterns Study (DOPPS). Am J Kidney Dis. 2013;62:738–46.

Chapter 13
Metabolic Acidosis and Progression of Chronic Kidney Disease

Csaba P. Kovesdy

Clinical Vignette

A 54-year-old African American male patient presents for initial evaluation of an elevated creatinine to the Nephrology outpatient clinic. He was referred by his primary care provider who detected a serum creatinine of 1.7 mg/dl on routine laboratory testing. The patient offers no particular subjective complaints. His past medical history includes hypertension diagnosed at age 41, controlled with medications since age 43. He is taking lisinopril 40 mg daily and amlodipine 5 mg daily. He denies using any over-the-counter medications or health supplements. His family history is significant for end stage kidney disease requiring dialysis in his mother and an uncle; the etiology of their kidney disease is unclear. The patient does not smoke, drinks alcohol socially less than once a month, and denies any illicit drug use. He works as an accountant, is married and has two children in college, none of whom have any chronic medical conditions. He tries to restrict salt intake in his diet. In his younger age he had been a vegetarian, but switched back to a meat-eating diet in the past few years. His physical exam shows a blood pressure of 132/74, a body mass index of 28 kg/m^2, and is otherwise unremarkable. Abnormal laboratory results included a serum creatinine of 1.8 mg/dl (corresponding to an estimated GFR of 48 ml/min/1.73 m^2 using the CKD-EPI formula), serum CO_2 (bicarbonate) of 22 mEq/l, blood hemoglobin of 13.2 g/dl, serum phosphorus of 4.6 mg/dl, serum parathyroid hormone of 128 pg/ml, a urinalysis showing 2+ protein on dipstick, and a random urine protein/creatinine ratio of 1254 mg/g. His kidney ultrasound is unremarkable except for increased echogenicity.

C.P. Kovesdy, M.D. (✉)
Division of Nephrology, University of Tennessee Health Science Center,
956 Court Avenue, Memphis, TN 38163, USA
e-mail: ckovesdy@uthsc.edu

© Springer Science+Business Media New York 2016
D.E. Wesson (ed.), *Metabolic Acidosis*, DOI 10.1007/978-1-4939-3463-8_13

Assessment

This patient presents with CKD, most likely caused by a genetic condition such as an APOL1 mutation. Clinical care of his CKD should include measures to prevent loss of kidney function, and management of metabolic conditions exacerbated by CKD. It is beyond the scope of this chapter to discuss all of these interventions; we will instead focus on addressing metabolic acidosis as it relates to progressive CKD and to interventions aimed at attenuating the loss of kidney function experienced by this patient.

Development of Metabolic Acidosis in CKD

Metabolic acidosis is a direct consequence of CKD. Kidney ammoniagenesis decreases early in the course of CKD because of decreasing numbers of functioning nephrons, in spite of a relative increase in single nephron ammoniagenesis [1]. In most patients the ability of the kidneys to maximally acidify urine and to reabsorb bicarbonate is maintained until very late stages of CKD [2, 3]. This kidney adaptation, combined with buffering that occurs most likely in the bone [4, 5] explains why most patients with even advanced CKD display only a mild metabolic acidosis with a normal or mildly widened anion gap. In addition, serum CO_2 levels are typically no lower than ~15 mEq/l [6, 7]. The role of CKD in engendering metabolic acidosis is also apparent in epidemiologic investigations which have shown that metabolic acidosis is increasingly common as kidney function worsens [8]. Most recently, in a population of over 570,000 US veterans the risk of metabolic acidosis was shown to increase linearly in patients with more advanced stages of CKD, especially in those with estimated GFR <45 ml/min/1.73 m^2 (Fig. 13.1) [9].

Consequences of Metabolic Acidosis

Maintaining a normal pH is important for the normal functioning of the human body. Depending on its severity, metabolic acidosis could have numerous adverse consequences, including osteopenia [4, 5], secondary hyperparathyroidism [10], reduced respiratory reserve, and exhaustion of body buffer systems which make patients more sensitive to the effects of acute illnesses [11], the reduction of Na^+-K^+-ATPase activity in red blood cells [12] and myocardial cells [13] which could lead to reduced myocardial contractility and congestive heart failure [14], abnormal glucose homeostasis, accumulation of beta-2 microglobulin, chronic inflammation, disturbances in growth hormone and thyroid function [15–17], the development of protein-energy wasting [17–22], increased cardiovascular events [23], and higher mortality [24–28]. However, more pertinent to the question of progressive CKD and to kidney protective therapies are the effects that metabolic acidosis have on the kidneys themselves.

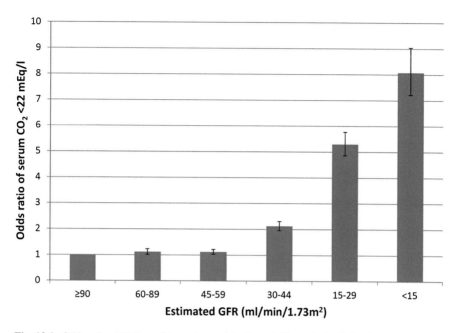

Fig. 13.1 Odds ratios (95 % confidence intervals) of metabolic acidosis (defined as proportion of patients with serum bicarbonate of <22 mEq/l) in a population-based cohort of 570,170 US veterans with non-dialysis dependent CKD stages 1–5, by CKD stage. Results are based on unpublished secondary analysis of data from Kovesdy et al. Circulation 2012 Feb 7;125(5):677–84 [75]

Several observational studies have indicated that lower serum CO_2 levels are associated with worse progression of CKD and a higher incidence of ESRD [23, 27, 29–32]. Due to their observational nature these studies could not conclude that metabolic acidosis is the actual cause of the worsened renal outcomes. Nevertheless, the plausibility of such a causal effect is bolstered by the growing basic science literature that has elucidated many of the mechanisms underlying the effect of metabolic acidosis on the kidney tissue and on kidney function (Fig. 13.2). One of the important adaptive kidney mechanisms against metabolic acidosis is ammonium production. Studies performed several decades ago have shown that ammonium production is associated with complement activation and increased tubulo-interstitial fibrosis, suggesting for the first time that chronic activation of adaptive mechanisms against metabolic acidosis could become maladaptive and lead to kidney injury [33–37]. A second important mechanism of kidney injury in metabolic acidosis was later suggested to be activation of endothelin production [38–42]. Enhanced distal nephron urinary acidification in response to an acid challenge to systemic acid–base status occurs through an endothelin-1 (ET-1)-dependent mechanism via activation of ET-B receptors. However, concomitant activation of ET-A receptors leads to interstitial fibrosis and progressive CKD [43–46]. Endothelin also activates aldosterone production, thus leading to further tubulo-interstitial damage [47]. Finally, metabolic acidosis directly activates the renin–angiotensin–aldosterone system, leading among others to further kidney damage [41, 42, 48–51].

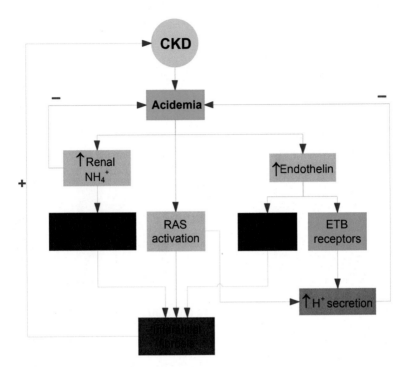

Fig. 13.2 Putative mechanisms of action of nephrotoxicity induced by metabolic acidosis. Adapted with permission from Kovesdy CP, Nephrol Dial Transplant (2012) 27: 3056–3062

Experimental studies suggest that interventions aimed at abrogating these pathways are beneficial in reducing kidney damage and delaying progression of CKD. These have included improvement in kidney histology [52], diminished kidney cyst formation and interstitial inflammation in a model of polycystic kidney disease [53, 54], and delayed progression of CKD [41] in animal experiments of bicarbonate administration. Early human studies have also shown improved biochemical and renal histological outcomes after bicarbonate administration in the face of metabolic acidosis [55, 56]. These studies have laid the foundation for clinical trials testing the hypothesis that chronic bicarbonate therapy could be applied as a renoprotective strategy and could lead to improved clinical end points in patients with CKD.

Alkali Therapy as an Effective Clinical Treatment of Progressive CKD

The plausibility of the metabolic acidosis-nephrotoxicity link is based on observational studies and compelling basic science findings. Nevertheless, in order to decisively prove the causal role of metabolic acidosis we need clinical trials showing that its treatment can alleviate kidney damage, leading to better renal outcomes. Besides proving the efficacy of therapeutic interventions, clinical trials are also needed to evaluate the safety of such interventions, and to define optimal therapeutic regimens that best balance risks and benefits.

The feasibility of alkali therapy as a renoprotective strategy was suggested by a small trial showing significant improvement in urinary markers of proximal tubular damage over 26 h in response to oral sodium bicarbonate in 11 patients with mild/moderate CKD and proteinuria [56], even though neither proteinuria, nor renal hemodynamics or systemic blood pressure were altered by the administration of sodium bicarbonate. Subsequently, moderately sized clinical trials have also corroborated the clinical benefit of alkali supplementation on progression of CKD (Table 13.1). In a single-center trial of 134 patients with advanced CKD (creatinine clearance 15–30 ml/min) and serum CO_2 of 16–20 mEq/l, oral bicarbonate therapy (titrated from a starting dose of 600 mg three times daily to achieve a serum CO_2 goal of 23 mEq/l) vs. placebo resulted in a lower rate of kidney function decline and a lower incidence of ESRD after 2 years [57]. Another study examined 59 patients with eGFR 20–60 ml/min/1.73 m² and baseline serum CO_2 of <22 mEq/l [55].

Table 13.1 Clinical trials of bicarbonate supplementation to prevent progression of CKD

Study	Population	Baseline serum CO_2	Therapy	Duration of intervention	Results
de Brito-Ashurst 2009 [57]	134 patients with creatinine clearance of 15–30 ml/min	16–20 mEq/l	Oral Na bicarbonate vs. open label standard care. Na bicarbonate titrated to achieve serum CO_2 >23 mEq/l	2 years	Decreased progression of CKD in the intervention arm: flatter slope, fewer rapid progressors, and fewer ESRD
Phisitkul 2010 [55]	59 patients with estimated GFR of 20–60 ml/min/1.73 m²	<22 mEq/l	Oral Na citrate vs. control	2 years	Decreased rate of progression in the Na citrate arm. Decreased urine endothelin and tubular injury markers in the Na citrate arm
Mahajan 2010 [58]	120 patients with estimated GFR 75±6 ml/min/1.73 m² and macroalbuminuria	≥24.5 mEq/l	Na bicarbonate vs. NaCl vs. placebo	5 years	Decreased rate of progression in the Na bicarbonate arm. Decreased urine endothelin and tubular injury markers in the Na bicarbonate arm. Decreased albuminuria in the Na bicarbonate arm

Patients were preference-randomized to 1 mEq of HCO_3 equivalent/kg body weight/ day sodium citrate in three divided doses (30 patients) vs. usual care (29 patients). The primary study end point was change in urine endothelin-1 levels; secondary end points were changes in urine markers of tubular damage and eGFR. After 24 months of therapy patients who received Na citrate displayed slower decline in kidney function, decreased urinary endothelin-1, decreased tubular injury markers, and decreased albuminuria. In a third study of 120 patients with hypertensive nephropathy with baseline eGFR of 75 ± 6 ml/min/1.73 m^2 and macroalbuminuria, and a serum bicarbonate level of at least 24.5 mEq/l, patients were randomized to oral Na bicarbonate (0.5 mEq/kg lean body weight/day) vs. oral NaCl (0.5 mEq/kg lean body weight/day) vs. placebo after matching for age, eGFR, albuminuria, and ethnicity [58]. The primary study end point was the reduction in the rate of eGFR decline after 5 years of follow-up; secondary end points were changes in urine endothelin, albuminuria, and markers of tubular injury. Patients who received sodium bicarbonate experienced significantly more favorable slopes of eGFR, decreases in urinary markers of tubular injury and urine endothelin, and stabilization of albuminuria. This study enrolled patients with early stage CKD and without manifest metabolic acidosis, supporting the notion that kidney protective interventions with oral alkali therapy could be applied preemptively at stages when kidney adaptive mechanisms are fully capable of maintaining the body's normal acid–base balance (vide supra).

Practical Considerations

Are We Using the Right Diagnostic Tools?

The above experimental studies suggest that the deleterious effect of metabolic acidosis on the kidneys is not necessarily induced by a low pH-mediated biochemical effect, but rather that it is mediated by the downstream effects of the numerous adaptive mechanisms the kidney uses to correct acidemia. The paradigm that chronic adaptive mechanisms over time become maladaptive and deleterious has important practical consequences for the optimal diagnosis of acidosis-related kidney damage. If a low pH is not a *condicio sine qua non* of metabolic acidosis-related chronic kidney damage, using a diagnostic approach based on proton retention and a consequent lowering of serum CO_2 may be missing a window of opportunity when acid–base homeostasis is maintained in balance by the above kidney adaptive mechanisms, but when kidney damage is already occurring as a result of these mechanisms.

It has been estimated that patients with frank metabolic acidosis (defined as a serum CO_2 concentration <22 mEq/l) may represent <10 % of the total CKD population [59], and hence restricting interventions of alkali therapy to this group may deprive a substantial group of patients from a potentially beneficial therapy. Direct measurement of one or more of the pathways responsible for acidosis-related damage could allow for earlier diagnosis and earlier therapy. This could involve assessment of increased urinary ammonium (or a surrogate marker of it, such as the urinary anion gap or urinary osmolar gap), or increased urinary endothelin levels. Levels of urinary endothelin have been shown to decrease after alkali therapy [55, 58], and hence this biomarker could also be used to monitor the effectiveness of therapeutic interventions. Notwithstanding the possibility that these tests will be used in the future in clinical practice, at the present time they are not widely available and there is also insufficient information on how they should be applied in practice (e.g., what are the normal ranges, and what cutoffs should trigger interventions?).

Due to the present practical difficulties with putative diagnostic markers, another potential approach would be to intervene with alkali therapy in every patient with CKD, not only those who have already developed frank metabolic acidosis. Proof of this concept was provided in a small single-center clinical trial (vide supra); but before its widespread application more investigation is needed to better delineate the upper boundaries of serum bicarbonate levels above which alkali administration could become deleterious (more on this later).

What Therapeutic Options Are There for the Treatment of Metabolic Acidosis?

The kidney damage induced by metabolic acidosis can in theory be alleviated by any measures that obviate the need for adaptive mechanisms aimed at enhancing kidney acid excretion. This can be achieved through the administration of sufficient base equivalents to buffer the amount of acids produced on a daily basis. Provided a typical western diet, an average person generates approximately 1 mEq of non-volatile acid/kg body weight/day [60]. Since a significant proportion of generated acid results from catabolism of nutrients containing proteins, one way to beneficially affect acid–base balance is through a diet composed of nutrients with a low acid load such as fruits and vegetables, e.g., a vegetarian diet [61]. Indeed, a recent study that compared a vegetarian diet with bicarbonate supplementation in patients with early CKD showed that the two approaches were equivalent in their ability to correct metabolic acidosis and to decrease biochemical markers of kidney injury [62]. Similar results were seen in a study that compared the two interventions in patients with advanced (stage 4) CKD [63]. Importantly, the dietary intervention did not result in the development of hyperkalemia in the study subjects who were selected to be at low risk for hyperkalemia, which is a significant concern in patients with advanced CKD receiving diets rich in vegetables and fruits. Whether such a dietary intervention is similarly safe outside of the strictly controlled confines of a clinical trial remains to be assessed individually. In addition to the benefits related to acid–base balance, a vegetarian diet could hold other important advantages to patients with CKD with direct effects on the progression of CKD [64], the discussion of which is beyond the scope of this chapter.

In patients who are unable or unwilling to change their dietary habits, or when administration of a more precise amount of bicarbonate is desired, medications containing bicarbonate or its equivalents (citrate or acetate) can be applied to buffer bodily acid production. Administration of these agents should be done with consideration for patients' individual characteristics to avoid any untoward consequences associated with either the bicarbonate component or the cation accompanying the bicarbonate moiety (or its equivalent). The amount administered depends on the desired therapeutic target, for which there is currently no uniform consensus yet. Of the most commonly used bicarbonate supplements, one 325 mg tablet of Na bicarbonate contains 4 mEq of bicarbonate, 1 ml of citric acid/trisodium citrate (Shohl's solution) contains 1 mEq of bicarbonate, and 1 ml of potassium citrate (Polycitra) contains 2 mEq of bicarbonate. The doses of these medications need to be titrated according to the desired serum CO_2 level. Professional guidelines recommend correction of metabolic acidosis (defined as a serum CO_2 <22 mEq/l) mainly because of its effects on protein-energy wasting [65]. However, one could argue that maintaining higher serum CO_2 levels and intervening even in patients who have not yet developed low serum CO_2 levels might provide clinical benefit (vide supra). Such a strategy would have to be implemented with proper safeguards to prevent potential deleterious consequences of bicarbonate administration, as will be discussed below.

Are There Any Deleterious Consequences of Alkali Therapy, and How to Avoid Them?

Observational studies suggest that the association of serum CO_2 levels with mortality is U-shaped, and abnormally high levels are also associated with adverse outcomes [24–26, 28]. These associations persisted even after adjustment for the typical comorbid conditions known to induce metabolic alkalosis (e.g., severe COPD, or chronic heart failure). Notwithstanding the possibility of residual confounding, metabolic alkalosis can have plausible direct adverse consequences. Acute effects of alkalemia include hypokalemia, hypocalcemia, or hypomagnesemia, with resultant cardiac arrhythmias [26, 66], which could explain the association of elevated serum CO_2 with increased mortality. There are also concerns about the effect of alkalemia on kidney function and kidney outcomes. Milk alkali syndrome is recognized as a consequence of alkalemia and high calcium intake, and can result in kidney damage and hastening of progressive CKD [67]. Under well-defined experimental circumstances higher bicarbonate resulted in renal calcium deposition in animals with elevated serum PO_4 levels, and metabolic acidosis had a protective effect [68–70]. Similar effects have not been described in humans, but caution may be advised in hyperphosphatemic patients receiving bicarbonate supplementation.

Besides the adverse consequences of CO_2 overloading, complications could arise as a result of mechanisms unrelated to changes in acid–base status. The administration of citrate-containing medications could enhance the absorption of aluminum from the gut, and could lead to aluminum-toxicity. It is thus recommended that patients with advanced CKD not receive their bicarbonate supplements in the form of citrate if they consume any aluminum-containing medications (such as various antacids). The administration of various cations that accompany the bicarbonate moiety or its equivalents could also have deleterious consequences. Ca-containing medications (such as Ca-acetate, Ca-carbonate, or Ca-citrate) could result in undesirably high calcium intake which has been linked to cardiovascular and soft tissue calcification in dialysis patients. Concerns have also been raised about the increased sodium intake resulting from Na bicarbonate supplements, which could hypothetically lead to volume overload, increased blood pressure, and adverse kidney and cardiovascular outcomes. These latter concerns have been alleviated by carefully conducted studies suggesting that the administration of Na bicarbonate has distinctly different effects compared to equivalent amounts of common salt (NaCl) [71–74], in that it does not result in substantial sodium retention, volume overload, and increased blood pressure.

In summary, potential adverse consequences of alkali administration are related to inadvertent induction of alkalemia, which could have acute and chronic complications related to kidney function and cardiovascular events. It is thus prudent to monitor serum CO_2 during therapy with bicarbonate, and withhold therapy when levels rise above the upper limit of the normal range. Sodium loading does not appear to be a problem with sodium bicarbonate administration. Other non-pH related adverse effects need to be addressed according to every patient's individual characteristics.

Management of the Clinical Case

Our patient presented with early stage CKD (stage 3A), and a borderline low serum CO_2 level. While he has yet to develop frank metabolic acidosis, it is likely that he has activated renal adaptive mechanisms to maintain normal acid–base balance. This could be confirmed by measuring a urine anion gap or a urine osmolar gap, although practically useable cutoffs for these tests have not been established yet for this indication. A more direct measure of activated kidney adaptive mechanism would be the level of urine endothelin, but this is not yet available for everyday clinical use. Alternatively, the patient could be treated empirically with a bicarbonate supplement, targeting a high-normal serum CO_2. Bicarbonate supplementation could be offered with a prescription medication titrated to the desired therapeutic goal, or the patient could revert to a vegetarian diet, if he feels motivated to do so. Either intervention would require monitoring of serum CO_2 levels to assure that therapeutic targets are met and that metabolic alkalosis does not develop, and of blood pressure and serum electrolytes, to assure optimization of kidney protection and prevention of potentially deleterious side effects (e.g., hyperkalemia or hyperphosphatemia).

Conclusions

Alterations in acid–base homeostasis happen with increasing frequency as CKD advances. The kidneys play a pivotal role in assuring that decreasing GFR does not result in acidemia, by activating redundant adaptive mechanisms that enhance acid excretion and assure a net even acid–base balance. Long-term activation of these adaptive mechanisms can, however, result in direct nephrotoxic effects, which is why metabolic acidosis is considered a causative factor for progressive kidney function loss. Several small clinical trials have shown that the administration of bicarbonate to patients with various stages of CKD is kidney protective. Due to the limitations of available evidence overarching recommendations regarding the indication of therapy, the best method(s) of bicarbonate replacement, the optimal therapeutic targets, and the likelihood of the efficacy and safety of such interventions cannot yet be made. Since bicarbonate supplementation is an affordable intervention which is likely safe and potentially beneficial, individualized treatment with various forms of bicarbonate or its equivalents should be considered in all patients with CKD who have no contraindication for such intervention.

References

1. Welbourne T, Weber M, Bank N. The effect of glutamine administration on urinary ammonium excretion in normal subjects and patients with renal disease. J Clin Invest. 1972;51(7): 1852–60.
2. Seldin DW, Coleman AJ, Carter NW, Rector Jr FC. The effect of Na_2SO_4 on urinary acidification in chronic renal disease. J Lab Clin Med. 1967;69(6):893–903.
3. Wong NL, Quamme GA, Dirks JH. Tubular handling of bicarbonate in dogs with experimental renal failure. Kidney Int. 1984;25(6):912–8.
4. Lemann Jr J, Litzow JR, Lennon EJ. The effects of chronic acid loads in normal man: further evidence for the participation of bone mineral in the defense against chronic metabolic acidosis. J Clin Invest. 1966;45(10):1608–14.
5. Green J, Kleeman CR. Role of bone in regulation of systemic acid–base balance. Kidney Int. 1991;39(1):9–26.
6. Widmer B, Gerhardt RE, Harrington JT, Cohen JJ. Serum electrolyte and acid base composition. The influence of graded degrees of chronic renal failure. Arch Intern Med. 1979;139(10):1099–102.
7. Hakim RM, Lazarus JM. Biochemical parameters in chronic renal failure. Am J Kidney Dis. 1988;11(3):238–47.
8. Eustace JA, Astor B, Muntner PM, Ikizler TA, Coresh J. Prevalence of acidosis and inflammation and their association with low serum albumin in chronic kidney disease. Kidney Int. 2004;65(3):1031–40.
9. Kovesdy CP. Metabolic acidosis and kidney disease: does bicarbonate therapy slow the progression of CKD? Nephrol Dial Transplant. 2012;27(8):3056–62.
10. Greenberg AJ, McNamara H, McCrory WW. Metabolic balance studies in primary renal tubular acidosis: effects of acidosis on external calcium and phosphorus balances. J Pediatr. 1966;69(4):610–8.
11. Tuso PJ, Nissenson AR, Danovitch GM. Electrolyte disorders in chronic renal failure. In: Narins RG, editor. Maxwell & Kleeman's clinical disorders of fluid and electrolyte metabolism. 5th ed. New York: McGraw-Hill, Inc.; 1994. p. 1195–211.
12. Levin ML, Rector Jr FC, Seldin DW. The effects of chronic hypokalaemia, hyponatraemia, and acid–base alterations on erythrocyte sodium transport. Clin Sci. 1972;43(2):251–63.
13. Brown Jr RH, Cohen I, Noble D. The interactions of protons, calcium and potassium ions on cardiac Purkinje fibres. J Physiol. 1978;282:345–52.
14. Mitchell JH, Wildenthal K, Johnson Jr RL. The effects of acid–base disturbances on cardiovascular and pulmonary function. Kidney Int. 1972;1(5):375–89.

15. Kopple JD, Kalantar-Zadeh K, Mehrotra R. Risks of chronic metabolic acidosis in patients with chronic kidney disease. Kidney Int Suppl. 2005;95:S21–7.
16. Kraut JA, Kurtz I. Metabolic acidosis of CKD: diagnosis, clinical characteristics, and treatment. Am J Kidney Dis. 2005;45(6):978–93.
17. Franch HA, Mitch WE. Catabolism in uremia: the impact of metabolic acidosis. J Am Soc Nephrol. 1998;9(12 Suppl):S78–81.
18. Mitch WE. Influence of metabolic acidosis on nutrition. Am J Kidney Dis. 1997;29(5):xlvi–xlviii.
19. Mitch WE, Du J, Bailey JL, Price SR. Mechanisms causing muscle proteolysis in uremia: the influence of insulin and cytokines. Miner Electrolyte Metab. 1999;25(4–6):216–9.
20. Ballmer PE, McNurlan MA, Hulter HN, Anderson SE, Garlick PJ, Krapf R. Chronic metabolic acidosis decreases albumin synthesis and induces negative nitrogen balance in humans. J Clin Invest. 1995;95(1):39–45.
21. Franch HA, Raissi S, Wang X, Zheng B, Bailey JL, Price SR. Acidosis impairs insulin receptor substrate-1-associated phosphoinositide 3-kinase signaling in muscle cells: consequences on proteolysis. Am J Physiol Renal Physiol. 2004;287(4):F700–6.
22. Uribarri J, Levin NW, Delmez J, Depner TA, Ornt D, Owen W, et al. Association of acidosis and nutritional parameters in hemodialysis patients. Am J Kidney Dis. 1999;34(3):493–9.
23. Dobre M, Yang W, Chen J, Drawz P, Hamm LL, Horwitz E, et al. Association of serum bicarbonate with risk of renal and cardiovascular outcomes in CKD: a report from the Chronic Renal Insufficiency Cohort (CRIC) study. Am J Kidney Dis. 2013.
24. Kovesdy CP, Anderson JE, Kalantar-Zadeh K. Association of serum bicarbonate levels with mortality in patients with non-dialysis-dependent CKD. Nephrol Dial Transplant. 2009;24(4):1232–7.
25. Bommer J, Locatelli F, Satayathum S, Keen ML, Goodkin DA, Saito A, et al. Association of predialysis serum bicarbonate levels with risk of mortality and hospitalization in the Dialysis Outcomes and Practice Patterns Study (DOPPS). Am J Kidney Dis. 2004;44(4):661–71.
26. Lowrie EG, Lew NL. Death risk in hemodialysis patients: the predictive value of commonly measured variables and an evaluation of death rate differences between facilities. Am J Kidney Dis. 1990;15(5):458–82.
27. Raphael KL, Wei G, Baird BC, Greene T, Beddhu S. Higher serum bicarbonate levels within the normal range are associated with better survival and renal outcomes in African Americans. Kidney Int. 2011;79(3):356–62.
28. Wu DY, McAllister CJ, Kilpatrick RD, Dadres S, Shinaberger CS, Kopple JD, et al. Association between serum bicarbonate and death in hemodialysis patients: is it better to be acidotic or alkalotic? Clin J Am Soc Nephrol. 2006;1:70–8.
29. Abramowitz MK, Melamed ML, Bauer C, Raff AC, Hostetter TH. Effects of oral sodium bicarbonate in patients with CKD. Clin J Am Soc Nephrol. 2013;8(5):714–20.
30. Kanda E, Ai M, Yoshida M, Kuriyama R, Shiigai T. High serum bicarbonate level within the normal range prevents the progression of chronic kidney disease in elderly chronic kidney disease patients. BMC Nephrol. 2013;14:4.
31. Scialla JJ, Appel LJ, Astor BC, Miller III ER, Beddhu S, Woodward M, et al. Net endogenous acid production is associated with a faster decline in GFR in African Americans. Kidney Int. 2012;82(1):106–12.
32. Shah SN, Abramowitz M, Hostetter TH, Melamed ML. Serum bicarbonate levels and the progression of kidney disease: a cohort study. Am J Kidney Dis. 2009;54(2):270–7.
33. Halperin ML, Ethier JH, Kamel KS. Ammonium excretion in chronic metabolic acidosis: benefits and risks. Am J Kidney Dis. 1989;14(4):267–71.
34. Nath KA, Hostetter MK, Hostetter TH. Pathophysiology of chronic tubulo-interstitial disease in rats. Interactions of dietary acid load, ammonia, and complement component C3. J Clin Invest. 1985;76(2):667–75.
35. Morita Y, Nomura A, Yuzawa Y, Nishikawa K, Hotta N, Shimizu F, et al. The role of complement in the pathogenesis of tubulointerstitial lesions in rat mesangial proliferative glomerulonephritis. J Am Soc Nephrol. 1997;8(9):1363–72.

36. Morita Y, Ikeguchi H, Nakamura J, Hotta N, Yuzawa Y, Matsuo S. Complement activation products in the urine from proteinuric patients. J Am Soc Nephrol. 2000;11(4):700–7.

37. Peake PW, Pussell BA, Mackinnon B, Charlesworth JA. The effect of pH and nucleophiles on complement activation by human proximal tubular epithelial cells. Nephrol Dial Transplant. 2002;17(5):745–52.

38. Wesson DE. Endogenous endothelins mediate increased distal tubule acidification induced by dietary acid in rats. J Clin Invest. 1997;99(9):2203–11.

39. Phisitkul S, Hacker C, Simoni J, Tran RM, Wesson DE. Dietary protein causes a decline in the glomerular filtration rate of the remnant kidney mediated by metabolic acidosis and endothelin receptors. Kidney Int. 2008;73(2):192–9.

40. Wesson DE, Nathan T, Rose T, Simoni J, Tran RM. Dietary protein induces endothelin-mediated kidney injury through enhanced intrinsic acid production. Kidney Int. 2007;71(3):210–7.

41. Wesson DE, Simoni J. Acid retention during kidney failure induces endothelin and aldosterone production which lead to progressive GFR decline, a situation ameliorated by alkali diet. Kidney Int. 2010;78(11):1128–35.

42. Wesson DE, Simoni J, Broglio K, Sheather S. Acid retention accompanies reduced GFR in humans and increases plasma levels of endothelin and aldosterone. Am J Physiol Renal Physiol. 2011;300(4):F830–7.

43. Khanna A, Simoni J, Hacker C, Duran MJ, Wesson DE. Increased endothelin activity mediates augmented distal nephron acidification induced by dietary protein. J Am Soc Nephrol. 2004;15(9):2266–75.

44. Wesson DE, Simoni J, Green DF. Reduced extracellular pH increases endothelin-1 secretion by human renal microvascular endothelial cells. J Clin Invest. 1998;101(3):578–83.

45. Wesson DE. Endogenous endothelins mediate increased acidification in remnant kidneys. J Am Soc Nephrol. 2001;12(9):1826–35.

46. Wesson DE. Regulation of kidney acid excretion by endothelins. Kidney Int. 2006;70(12):2066–73.

47. Khanna A, Simoni J, Wesson DE. Endothelin-induced increased aldosterone activity mediates augmented distal nephron acidification as a result of dietary protein. J Am Soc Nephrol. 2005;16(7):1929–35.

48. Ng HY, Chen HC, Tsai YC, Yang YK, Lee CT. Activation of intrarenal renin-angiotensin system during metabolic acidosis. Am J Nephrol. 2011;34(1):55–63.

49. Wesson DE, Jo CH, Simoni J. Angiotensin II receptors mediate increased distal nephron acidification caused by acid retention. Kidney Int. 2012;82(11):1184–94.

50. Goraya N, Simoni J, Jo CH, Wesson DE. Treatment of metabolic acidosis in patients with stage 3 chronic kidney disease with fruits and vegetables or oral bicarbonate reduces urine angiotensinogen and preserves glomerular filtration rate. Kidney Int. 2014;86:1031–8.

51. Wesson DE, Jo CH, Simoni J. Angiotensin II-mediated GFR decline in subtotal nephrectomy is due to acid retention associated with reduced GFR. Nephrol Dial Transplant. 2014.

52. Gadola L, Noboa O, Marquez MN, Rodriguez MJ, Nin N, Boggia J, et al. Calcium citrate ameliorates the progression of chronic renal injury. Kidney Int. 2004;65(4):1224–30.

53. Torres VE, Mujwid DK, Wilson DM, Holley KH. Renal cystic disease and ammoniagenesis in Han: SPRD rats. J Am Soc Nephrol. 1994;5(5):1193–200.

54. Torres VE, Cowley Jr BD, Branden MG, Yoshida I, Gattone VH. Long-term ammonium chloride or sodium bicarbonate treatment in two models of polycystic kidney disease. Exp Nephrol. 2001;9(3):171–80.

55. Phisitkul S, Khanna A, Simoni J, Broglio K, Sheather S, Rajab MH, et al. Amelioration of metabolic acidosis in patients with low GFR reduced kidney endothelin production and kidney injury, and better preserved GFR. Kidney Int. 2010;77(7):617–23.

56. Rustom R, Grime JS, Costigan M, Maltby P, Hughes A, Taylor W, et al. Oral sodium bicarbonate reduces proximal renal tubular peptide catabolism, ammoniogenesis, and tubular damage in renal patients. Ren Fail. 1998;20(2):371–82.

57. de Brito-Ashurst I, Varagunam M, Raftery MJ, Yaqoob MM. Bicarbonate supplementation slows progression of CKD and improves nutritional status. J Am Soc Nephrol. 2009;20(9):2075–84.

58. Mahajan A, Simoni J, Sheather SJ, Broglio KR, Rajab MH, Wesson DE. Daily oral sodium bicarbonate preserves glomerular filtration rate by slowing its decline in early hypertensive nephropathy. Kidney Int. 2010;78(3):303–9.
59. Kovesdy CP, Kalantar-Zadeh K. Oral bicarbonate: renoprotective in CKD? Nat Rev Nephrol. 2010;6(1):15–7.
60. Moe OW, Rector FC, Alpern RJ. Renal regulation of acid–base metabolism. In: Narins RG, editor. Maxwell and Kleeman's clinical disorders of fluid and electrolyte metabolism. 5th ed. New York: McGraw-Hill, Inc.; 1994. p. 203–42.
61. Remer T, Manz F. Potential renal acid load of foods and its influence on urine pH. J Am Diet Assoc. 1995;95(7):791–7.
62. Goraya N, Simoni J, Jo C, Wesson DE. Dietary acid reduction with fruits and vegetables or bicarbonate attenuates kidney injury in patients with a moderately reduced glomerular filtration rate due to hypertensive nephropathy. Kidney Int. 2012;81(1):86–93.
63. Goraya N, Simoni J, Jo CH, Wesson DE. A comparison of treating metabolic acidosis in CKD stage 4 hypertensive kidney disease with fruits and vegetables or sodium bicarbonate. Clin J Am Soc Nephrol. 2013;8(3):371–81.
64. Kovesdy CP, Kopple JD, Kalantar-Zadeh K. Management of protein-energy wasting in non-dialysis-dependent chronic kidney disease: reconciling low protein intake with nutritional therapy. Am J Clin Nutr. 2013;97(6):1163–77.
65. National Kidney Foundation. K/DOQI clinical practice guidelines for nutrition in chronic renal failure. Am J Kidney Dis. 2000;35(6 Suppl 1):s1–140.
66. Kovesdy CP, Regidor DL, Mehrotra R, Jing J, McAllister CJ, Greenland S, et al. Serum and dialysate potassium concentrations and survival in hemodialysis patients. Clin J Am Soc Nephrol. 2007;2(5):999–1007.
67. Felsenfeld AJ, Levine BS. Milk alkali syndrome and the dynamics of calcium homeostasis. Clin J Am Soc Nephrol. 2006;1(4):641–54.
68. Jara A, Felsenfeld AJ, Bover J, Kleeman CR. Chronic metabolic acidosis in azotemic rats on a high-phosphate diet halts the progression of renal disease. Kidney Int. 2000;58(3):1023–32.
69. Jara A, Chacon C, Ibaceta M, Valdivieso A, Felsenfeld AJ. Effect of ammonium chloride and dietary phosphorus in the azotemic rat. I. Renal function and biochemical changes. Nephrol Dial Transplant. 2004;19(8):1986–92.
70. Jara A, Chacon C, Ibaceta M, Valdivieso A, Felsenfeld AJ. Effect of ammonium chloride and dietary phosphorus in the azotaemic rat. Part II—Kidney hypertrophy and calcium deposition. Nephrol Dial Transplant. 2004;19(8):1993–8.
71. Husted FC, Nolph KD, Maher JF. NaHCO$_3$ and NaCl tolerance in chronic renal failure. J Clin Invest. 1975;56(2):414–9.
72. Husted FC, Nolph KD. NaHCO$_3$ and NaCl tolerance in chronic renal failure II. Clin Nephrol. 1977;7(1):21–5.
73. Luft FC, Zemel MB, Sowers JA, Fineberg NS, Weinberger MH. Sodium bicarbonate and sodium chloride: effects on blood pressure and electrolyte homeostasis in normal and hypertensive man. J Hypertens. 1990;8(7):663–70.
74. Wesson DE. Glomerular filtration effects of acute volume expansion: importance of chloride. Kidney Int. 1987;32(2):238–45.
75. Kovesdy CP, Lott EH, Lu JL, Malakauskas SM, Ma JZ, Molnar MZ, et al. Hyponatremia, hypernatremia, and mortality in patients with chronic kidney disease with and without congestive heart failure. Circulation. 2012;125(5):677–84.

Chapter 14
Management of Chronic Metabolic Acidosis

Donald E. Wesson

Introduction

Chronic metabolic acidosis is a common disorder which, even when "mild," is associated with untoward complications including increased mortality as detailed elsewhere in this book. It is a common complication of chronic kidney disease (CKD), an increasing health burden [1]. Renal tubular acidoses are another form of chronic metabolic acidosis and can be idiopathic in presentation or a component of systemic diseases like lupus which adversely affect kidney tubule function. Consequently, chronic metabolic acidosis will continue to exact a toll on patients and continue to challenge clinicians with its management into the foreseeable future.

Acute metabolic acidosis is most commonly seen in critically ill inpatients. Its treatment is discussed in detail elsewhere in this book but in general, it is best treated by correcting the underlying disorder leading to metabolic acidosis. Selected patients might benefit from $NaHCO_3$ administration but these benefits must be weighed against the risks associated with this intervention in some critically ill patients.

Metabolic acidosis is a process characterized by net gain of hydrogen ion (H^+) and/or loss of base (usually HCO_3). It is manifest in laboratory data by a decrease in serum $[HCO_3]$ and a physiologic response of increased ventilation reflected by decreased partial pressure of carbon dioxide (PCO_2). Body systems can prevent or mitigate metabolic acidosis in response to H^+ gain or HCO_3 loss by using buffers to minimize pH/$[HCO_3]$ changes in response to the acid challenge, or by kidney excretion of added H^+ that regenerates HCO_3 to replace HCO_3 titrated by the added H^+ (see Fig. 14.1). Kidneys require a few days to excrete sufficient H^+ to regenerate new HCO_3 to replace acute HCO_3 losses.

D.E. Wesson, M.D., M.B.A. (✉)
Baylor Scott and White Health, Department of Internal Medicine, Texas A&M Health
Sciences Center College of Medicine, 2401 South 31st Street, Temple, TX 76508, USA
e-mail: dwesson@sw.org

© Springer Science+Business Media New York 2016   145
D.E. Wesson (ed.), *Metabolic Acidosis*, DOI 10.1007/978-1-4939-3463-8_14

General Causes of Metabolic Acidosis

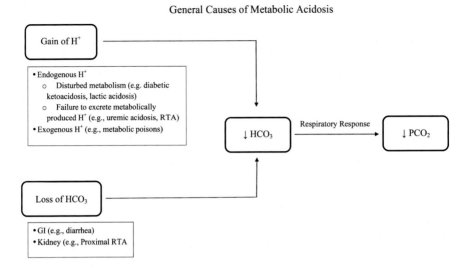

Fig. 14.1 General causes of metabolic acidosis

Metabolic acidosis might therefore occur because (1) the magnitude of added H^+ or lost HCO_3 overwhelms normal buffering and/or normal kidney H^+ excretory capacity; (2) buffering capacity is compromised; and/or (3) kidney H^+ excretory capacity is compromised or has had insufficient time to replace acutely lost HCO_3. In most settings clinicians have little opportunity to improve body buffering or increase kidney excretory capacity to "correct" metabolic acidosis. Consequently, clinicians' most common tool to treat metabolic acidosis is to administer base and/or decrease dietary acid.

Current kidney community guidelines recommend treating chronic metabolic acidosis associated with CKD by increasing dietary base using Na^+ citrate or $NaHCO_3$ and doing so only for patients with serum total CO_2 (TCO_2)<22 mM [2]. Nevertheless, the risk for mortality, adverse cardiovascular outcomes, and the rate of GFR decline increases in CKD patients as serum TCO_2 decreases due to metabolic acidosis within ranges that include values >22 mM and even into the normal range [3–6]. Animal models of CKD with reduced GFR but no metabolic acidosis nevertheless have tissue H^+ retention [7, 8] and patients with reduced eGFR without metabolic acidosis might also have H^+ retention [9]. In addition, oral K^+HCO_3 improved mineral balance and skeletal metabolism in post-menopausal women not known to have metabolic acidosis [10]. Future studies will determine if dietary H^+ reduction benefits patients without depressed GFR but who are ingesting the high H^+ diets of industrialized societies [11] and/or benefits patients with depressed GFR but without metabolic acidosis.

Diets in industrialized societies are largely H^+-producing when metabolized [11] and dietary addition of base-producing fruits and vegetables (F + V) reduces urine net acid excretion (NAE) [12] consistent with reduced net endogenous H^+ production [13]. In addition, F + V improve metabolic acidosis in CKD [14, 15] and so are a treatment option for chronic metabolic acidosis due to CKD and possibly other disorders of chronic metabolic acidosis. Furthermore, high dietary H^+ can induce metabolic acidosis in patients with low GFR but lower H^+ diets might not cause metabolic acidosis in these same patients [16]. These data point out the importance of dietary H^+ in patients with reduced GFR, particularly the elderly [13] and support dietary H^+ reduction as an effective treatment strategy for metabolic acidosis.

Response to an Acid Challenge

Dietary H^+ challenges cause directional increases in serum $[H^+]$ (decreases in pH) with directional decreases in serum $[HCO_3]$ but quantitatively large changes in dietary H^+ yield quantitatively small changes in $[H^+]/[HCO_3]$ [17]. Additionally, even large changes in dietary H^+ elicit serum $[H^+]/[HCO_3]$ changes that typically fall within the normal range for each [17] so measuring serum $[H^+]/[HCO_3]$ typically provides little insight as to the magnitude of dietary H^+ or base. These data attest to the effectiveness of body buffers and kidney excretory capacity to maintain serum $[H^+]/[HCO_3]$. On the other hand, patients with reduced baseline GFR can have greater increases in $[H^+]$ and greater decreases in $[HCO_3]$ in response to dietary H^+ challenges, even developing metabolic acidosis in response to H^+ challenges that do not cause metabolic acidosis in patients with higher GFR [16]. Consequently, clinicians are more likely to recognize metabolic acidosis in patients with lower compared to higher GFR.

Because the increment in kidney H^+ excretion in response to an increment in dietary H^+ is less than the increment in dietary H^+, even in individuals with normal baseline GFR, increments in dietary H^+ appear to induce H^+ retention [18]. Because this apparent H^+ retention is typically accompanied by only minor increases in serum $[H^+]$ and only minor decreases in serum $[HCO_3]$ as indicated earlier [17], much of this retained H^+ titrates body buffers. Animal studies support that this H^+ retention is greater with reduced compared to normal GFR [7, 8]. Because $KHCO_3$ preserves bone mineral content in patients with normal GFR [10] and because $NaHCO_3$ preserves eGFR in patients with reduced GFR but not metabolic acidosis [19] who nevertheless appear to have H^+ retention [9], underlying H^+ retention in the absence of metabolic acidosis by serum acid–base parameters might have untoward effects that can be ameliorated through dietary H^+ reduction. Future studies will test this hypothesis.

Types of Chronic Metabolic Acidoses for Which Treatment Should Be Considered

Because of its untoward consequences described elsewhere in this book, chronic metabolic acidosis, even when mild, should be treated.

Renal Tubule Acidoses

Proximal Renal Tubule Acidosis Patients with proximal renal tubule acidosis (PRTA) have defective proximal tubule HCO_3 reabsorption with excess terminal nephron HCO_3 delivery that overwhelms capacity of the distal nephron to completely reabsorb the high HCO_3 delivered load. Because urine NAE = urine ammonium + urine titratable acidity − urine HCO_3, excess urine HCO_3 excretion reduces urine NAE. These patients reach a steady-state of chronically low serum [HCO_3] at which the defective proximal tubule more completely reabsorbs the lower amount of HCO_3 filtered into the nephron (because of lower serum [HCO_3]). This lower HCO_3 delivery to the terminal nephron allows the functionally intact distal nephron to effectively excrete ammonium and titratable acidity without excess urine HCO_3 excretion. This steady-state scenario allows the kidney to maintain net acid balance, i.e., match dietary intake with that excreted. The steady-state price paid is that these patients have chronic metabolic acidosis manifest by low serum [HCO_3] (with a physiologic response to decrease PCO_2).

The most concerning consequence of the chronic metabolic acidosis of PRTA is the inhibited bone growth in children [20]. The chronic metabolic acidosis is also associated with low bone mineral content as rickets in children and osteomalacia in adults and nephrolithiasis in both [21]. Treatment of metabolic acidosis in PRTA with large volumes of $NaHCO_3$, typically 10–15 meq/kg body weight/day [20, 21], is needed to maintain serum [HCO_3] at a high enough level to avoid or ameliorate these untoward consequences. Such treatment leads to large urine HCO_3 losses that obligate potassium and phosphate losses that also require replacement [20]. The large alkali requirements of patients with PRTA cannot be met with only reducing acid-producing and/or adding base-producing dietary constituents.

Distal Renal Tubule Acidosis Patients with distal renal tubule acidosis (DRTA) have intact proximal tubule function and so do not deliver large HCO_3 loads to the terminal nephron. In contrast with PRTA, these patients have defective distal nephron acidification such that they have lower excretion of ammonium and/or titratable acidity [22, 23]. Consequently, patients with DRTA are typically unable to completely excrete the standard dietary acid load ingested by members of industrialized societies and so are in steady-state net acid retention without treatment [23]. The acid retained lowers serum [HCO_3] (with a physiologic response to decrease PCO_2) and so these patients have chronic metabolic acidosis. The net acid retention causes bone disease and nephrolithiasis [21, 24].

Because patients with DRTA have intact proximal tubule function, they do not have the large urine HCO_3 losses of PRTA and so do not have the large alkali requirements of PRTA patients. Instead, DRTA patients require alkali sufficient to treat the described net acid retention. Individuals in industrialized societies typically ingest diets that produce about 1–1.5 meq/kg body weight/day net of acid [25] and so most recommendations suggest that DRTA patients receive as much alkali daily, typically as NaHCO$_3$ [23]. Although there are no published studies describing DRTA treatment exclusively by reducing acid-producing or adding base-producing dietary constituents, the comparatively lower alkali requirements of patients with DRTA suggest that dietary strategies might be used at least as adjunctive treatment to Na$^+$ or K$^+$-based alkali.

Chronic Metabolic Acidosis of Chronic Kidney Disease

The 2013 KDIGO guidelines [2] are the most carefully prescribed recommendations for treatment of chronic metabolic acidosis but it is not clear that these recommendations should be applied unmodified to other etiologies of chronic metabolic acidosis. These recommendations read as follows: "We suggest that in people with CKD and serum bicarbonate concentrations <22 mmol/l treatment with oral bicarbonate supplementation be given to maintain serum bicarbonate within the normal range, unless contraindicated." The authors comment that the indicated serum [HCO$_3$] below which to treat has not been rigorously determined with large-scale studies but reflects opinions and experience of the authors. Recommended doses range from 0.5 to 1.0 meq HCO$_3$ or its equivalent per kg lean body weight daily. This is similar in amount to that recommended for DRTA because the concern with the chronic metabolic acidosis of CKD is the failure to completely excrete metabolically produced acid, mostly from dietary intake. The treatment goal, as stated in KDIGO, is to maintain serum HCO$_3$ in the normal range. The guidelines recommend Na$^+$-based alkali therapy such as Na$^+$ citrate or NaHCO$_3$ as tolerated.

General Management Strategies for Metabolic Acidosis

Increase H$^+$ Removal (Enhanced GFR or Dialysis)

Some patients with acute kidney injury (AKI) develop metabolic acidosis because of their temporary reduction in GFR and/or because the GFR reduction was so acute that the remaining functioning nephrons did not have time to increase per nephron acidification as seen in experimental animals with chronic GFR reduction [26]. If clinical interventions allow restoration of normal GFR or improved GFR above the present low level, kidney H$^+$ excretory capacity can increase to levels sufficient to improve or even completely correct underlying metabolic acidosis. If, however, clinicians surmise that GFR will not recover or its recovery is not eminent, dialysis might be instituted to remove H$^+$ from body fluids and add HCO$_3$ from dialysate to treat the metabolic acidosis.

Improve Body Buffering Capacity

Added H^+ to body fluids is buffered predominantly intracellularly [25, 27] with most extracellular buffering done by hemoglobin [28] with lesser contribution from albumin [28, 29]. Although clinicians might theoretically increase body buffering capacity by increasing blood hemoglobin or serum albumin, these measures have little quantitative impact.

Dietary H^+ Reduction

Na^+-Based Alkali Therapies Sodium bicarbonate ($NaHCO_3$) is the common alkali salt used to treat metabolic acidosis because it is effective, relatively well-tolerated, widely available, and inexpensive. Potassium bicarbonate is used less commonly, except in patients who require substantial HCO_3 replacement (like PRTA) that is associated with large K^+ losses in response to treatment. Potassium bicarbonate should be avoided in patients with very low GFR (<25 % of normal) because of the risk for K^+ retention with hyperkalemia. Because citrate is metabolized to yield HCO_3, Na^+ citrate is often used in patients unable to tolerate K^+. Use of Na^+ citrate is limited by its unpleasant taste, comparatively high expense, and because it promotes gastric aluminum absorption [30]. Consequently, $NaHCO_3$ is the alkali salt upon which we will focus our discussion.

Oral $NaHCO_3$ rapidly reacts with gastric hydrochloric acid (HCl) to form NaCl, CO_2, and H_2O. Excess HCO_3 that does not neutralize gastric acid rapidly empties into the small intestine and is absorbed. Reaction of $NaHCO_3$ with gastric HCl increases gastric lumen pH, stimulating gastric parietal cells to secrete more HCl into the gastric lumen. Secretion of HCl into the gastric lumen induced by the rise in gastric pH leads to HCO_3 extrusion into peri-gastric capillaries and eventually into the systemic circulation to increase ECF HCO_3 if it is reduced. Extracellular HCO_3 that exceeds the kidney tubule maximum for reabsorption is eliminated in the urine.

Orally administered $NaHCO_3$ has had few notable side effects when given to CKD patients [19, 31–34]. Most side effects from $NaHCO_3$ were caused by release of CO_2 gas when it contacts gastric H^+ and consists of belching, gastric distension, and flatus. Higher doses might theoretically cause volume retention and possibly exacerbate hypertension in patients with very low GFR. Nevertheless, studies in which $NaHCO_3$ was administered to CKD patients at much higher than the recommended KDIGO doses showed that $NaHCO_3$ did not increase blood pressure or cause edema [35]. Because serum alkalization decreases ionized calcium, HCO_3 therapy or its equivalent might theoretically cause tissue, importantly vascular, calcification. Indeed, both calcium containing and non-calcium containing alkali salts have been associated with progressive (but not de novo) vessel calcification [36]. On the other hand, $NaHCO_3$ therapy did not change serum total calcium and inorganic phosphorus concentrations or the calcium/phosphate product in CKD patients [37]. Consequently, more studies will determine if the described benefits of bicarbonate therapy in CKD patients with metabolic acidosis are counterbalanced by untoward effects of progressive and/or de novo vascular calcification.

Adding Base-Inducing Dietary Components High dietary H^+ contributes to metabolic acidosis in patients with reduced GFR [16]. Consequently, dietary H^+ reduction might be accomplished by adding or substituting base-inducing foods like fruits and vegetables to the high H^+ diet typical of industrialized societies. Acid contents of many foods have been published [38] and might be used to determine how much of what foods to prescribe to CKD patients. Adding base-producing fruits and vegetables reduced urine NAE in CKD patients with reduced eGFR but no metabolic acidosis [12] and also improved metabolic acidosis in CKD patients whose eGFR was low enough to be associated with metabolic acidosis [14, 15, 39]. In these studies [12, 14, 15], fruits and vegetables were prescribed in amounts equivalent to 50 % of their calculated dietary H^+ load. For most patients, this amounted to adding 2–3 cups of fruits and vegetables to their daily diets. Patient participants in these studies were carefully selected to be at very low risk to develop hyperkalemia in response to the increased K^+ load that accompanies fruits and vegetables. Therefore, clinicians should use caution when considering prescribing fruits and vegetables to CKD patients, particularly those with very low GFR.

Conclusion

Metabolic acidosis is common, appears to contribute to increase mortality, and contributes to morbidity such as decreased bone mineral content, increased protein catabolism, and possibly enhanced nephropathy progression in CKD. These data highlight the need to treat this syndrome that continues to increase in prevalence [1]. Most of these untoward consequences of metabolic acidosis can be mitigated by treating metabolic acidosis and so clinicians have an imperative to do so. The most effective mechanism to treat metabolic acidosis available to clinicians is dietary H^+ reduction that can be accomplished with Na^+-based alkali and/or with base-producing food components like fruits and vegetables. Each of these strategies to reduce dietary H^+ is relatively inexpensive and comparatively well-tolerated. Whether CKD patients with reduced GFR but no metabolic acidosis or selected patients with normal GFR but eating diets of high H^+ content are candidates for dietary H^+ reduction will be determined by further study.

Conflict of Interest Statement The author has no conflicts to report.

References

1. US Burden of Disease Collaborators. The state of US health, 1990–2010. Burden of diseases, injuries, and risk factors. JAMA. 2013;310:591–608.
2. KDIGO Guidelines. Chapter 3: management of progression and complications of CKD. Kidney Int. 2013;Suppl 3:73–90.
3. Kovesdy CP, Anderson JE, Kalantar-Zadeh K. Association of serum bicarbonate levels with mortality in patients with non-dialysis-dependent CKD. Nephrol Dial Transplant. 2009;24:1232–7.
4. Raphael K, Wei G, Baird B, et al. Higher plasma bicarbonate levels within the normal range are associated with better survival and renal outcomes in African Americans. Kidney Int. 2011;79:356–62.
5. Shah SN, Abramowitz M, Hostetter TH, et al. Plasma bicarbonate levels and the progression of kidney disease: a cohort study. Am J Kidney Dis. 2009;54:270–7.
6. Dobre MD, Yang W, Chen J, et al. Association of plasma bicarbonate with risk of renal and cardiovascular outcomes in CKD: a report from the chronic renal insufficiency cohort (CRIC) study. Am J Kidney Dis. 2013;62:670–8.
7. Wesson DE, Simoni J. Increased tissue acid mediates progressive GFR decline in animals with reduced nephron mass. Kidney Int. 2009;75:929–35.
8. Wesson DE, Simoni J. Acid retention during kidney failure induces endothelin and aldosterone production which lead to progressive GFR decline, a situation ameliorated by alkali diet. Kidney Int. 2010;78:1128–35.
9. Wesson DE, Simoni J, Broglio K, Sheather S. Acid retention accompanies reduced GFR in humans and increases plasma levels of endothelin and aldosterone. Am J Physiol Renal Physiol. 2011;300:F830–7.
10. Sebastian A, Harris ST, Ottaway JH, Todd KM, Morris Jr RC. Improved mineral balance and skeletal metabolism in postmenopausal women treated with potassium bicarbonate. N Engl J Med. 1994;330:1776–81.
11. Remer T. Influence of nutrition on acid-base balance-metabolic aspects. Eur J Nutr. 2001;40:214–20.
12. Goraya N, Simoni J, Jo C-H, Wesson DE. Dietary acid reduction with fruits and vegetables or sodium bicarbonate reduces kidney injury in individuals with moderately reduced GFR due to hypertensive nephropathy. Kidney Int. 2011;81:86–93.
13. Frassetto LA, Todd K, Morris Jr RC, Sebastian A. Estimation of net endogenous noncarbonic acid production in humans from diet potassium and protein contents. Am J Clin Nutr. 1998;68:576–83.
14. Goraya N, Simoni J, Jo C-H, Wesson DE. Comparison of treating the metabolic acidosis of CKD stage 4 hypertensive kidney disease with fruits and vegetables or sodium bicarbonate. Clin J Am Soc Nephrol. 2013;8:371–81.
15. Goraya N, Simoni J, Jo C-H, Wesson DE. Treatment of metabolic acidosis in individuals with stage 3 CKD with fruits and vegetables or oral NaHCO3 reduces urine angiotensinogen and preserves GFR. Kidney Int. 2014;86:1031–8.
16. Adeva MM, Souto G. Diet-induced metabolic acidosis. Clin Nutr. 2011;30:416–21.
17. Kurtz I, Maher T, Hulter HN, et al. Effect of diet on plasma acid-base composition in normal humans. Kidney Int. 1983;24:670–80.
18. Lemann Jr J, Bushinsky DA, Hamm LL. Bone buffering of acid and base in humans. Am J Physiol Renal Physiol. 2003;285:F811–32.
19. Mahajan A, Simoni J, Sheather S, Broglio K, Rajab MH, Wesson DE. Daily oral sodium bicarbonate preserves glomerular filtration rate by slowing its decline in early hypertensive nephropathy. Kidney Int. 2010;78:303–9.
20. McSherry E. Renal tubular acidosis in childhood. Kidney Int. 1981;20:799–809.
21. Brenner RJ, Spring DB, Sebastian A, McSherry EM, Palubinskas AJ, Morris Jr RC. Incidence of radiographically evident bone disease, nephrocalcinosis, and nephrolithiasis in various types of renal tubular acidosis. N Engl J Med. 1982;307:217–21.

22. Caruana RJ, Buckalew Jr VM. The syndrome of distal (type 1) renal tubular acidosis. Clinical and laboratory findings in 58 cases. Medicine (Baltimore). 1988;67:84–99.
23. Kurtzman NA. Disorders of distal acidification. Kidney Int. 1990;38:720–7.
24. Coe FL, Parks JH. Stone disease in hereditary distal renal tubular acidosis. Ann Intern Med. 1980;93:60–61.
25. Goodman AD, Lemann Jr J, Lennon EJ, Relman AS. Production, excretion, and net balance of fixed acid in patients with renal failure. J Clin Invest. 1980;17:595–606.
26. Wesson DE, Jo C-H, Simoni J. Animals with reduced GFR but no metabolic acidosis nevertheless have increased distal nephron acidification that is induced by acid retention and mediated through angiotensin II receptors. Kidney Int. 2012;82:1184–94.
27. Schwartz WB, Orning KJ, Porter R. The internal distribution of hydrogen ions with varying degrees of metabolic acidosis. J Clin Invest. 1957;36:373–82.
28. Kancir CB, Petersen PH, Madsen T. Effects of erythrocytes, bicarbonate, temperature, and albumin on in vitro ionized calcium variations with pH. Scand J Clin Lab Invest. 1989;49:475–82.
29. Levraut J, Garcia P, Giunti C, Ichai C, Bouregba M, Ciebiera JP, Payan P, Grimaud D. The increase in CO2 production induced by NaHCO3 depends on blood albumin and hemoglobin concentrations. Intensive Care Med. 2000;26:558–64.
30. Nolan C, Califano JR, Butzin CA. Influence of calcium acetate or calcium citrate on intestinal aluminum absorption. Kidney Int. 1990;38:937–41.
31. de Brito-Ashurst I, Varagunam M, Raferty MJ, Yaqoob M. Bicarbonate supplementation slows progression of CKD and improves nutritional status. J Am Soc Nephrol. 2009;20:2075–84.
32. Susantitaphong P, Sewaralthahab K, Balk EM, et al. Short- and long-term effects of alkali therapy in chronic kidney disease: a systematic review. Am J Nephrol. 2012;35:540–7.
33. Abramowitz MK, Melamed ML, Bauer C, et al. Effects of oral sodium bicarbonate on patients with CKD. Clin J Am Soc Nephrol. 2013;8:714–20.
34. Loniewski I, Wesson DE. Bicarbonate therapy for kidney disease. Kidney Int. 2014;85:529–35.
35. Husted FC, Nolph KD. NaHCO3 and NaCl tolerance in chronic renal failure. Clin Nephrol. 1977;7:21–5.
36. Block GA, Wheeler DC, Persky MS, et al. Effects of phosphate binders in moderate CKD. J Am Soc Nephrol. 2012;23:1407–15.
37. Mathur RP, Dash SC, Gupta N, et al. Effects of correction of metabolic acidosis on blood urea and bone metabolism in patients with mild to moderate chronic kidney disease: a prospective randomized single blind controlled trial. Ren Fail. 2006;28:1–5.
38. Remer T, Manz F. Potential renal acid load of foods and its influence on urine pH. J Am Diet Assoc. 1995;95:791–7.
39. Barsotti G, Morelli E, Cupisti A, Meola M, Dani L, Giovannetti S. A low-nitrogen low phosphorous vegan diet for patients with chronic renal failure. Nephron. 1996;74:390–4.

Index